OBSTETRICAL PEARLS

A PRACTICAL GUIDE FOR THE EFFICIENT RESIDENT

OBSTETRICAL PEARLS

A PRACTICAL GUIDE
FOR THE
EFFICIENT RESIDENT

Second Edition

MICHAEL D. BENSON, MD, FACOG
Lecturer
Department of Obstetrics
and Gynecology
Northwestern University
Medical School
Chicago, Illinois

 F. A. Davis Company • Philadelphia

F. A. Davis Company
1915 Arch Street
Philadelphia, PA 19103

Copyright © 1994 by F. A. Davis Company

Printed in Canada

Last digit indicates print number: 10 9 8 7 6 5 4 3 2 1

Medical Editor: Robert W. Reinhardt
Medical Developmental Editor: Bernice M. Wissler
Production Editor: Crystal S. McNichol
Cover Design By: Donald B. Freggens, Jr.

Library of Congress Cataloging-in-Publication Data

Benson, Michael D.
    Obstetrical pearls : a practical guide for the efficient resident / Michael D. Benson. — 2nd ed.
        p. cm.
    Includes index.
    ISBN 0-8036-0702-4 (softback : alk. paper)
    1. Obstetrics—Handbooks, manuals, etc. I. Title.
    [DNLM: 1. Obstetrics—handbooks. 2. Pregnancy Complications—handbooks. WQ 39 B474o 1994]
    RG531.B46 1994
    618.2—dc20
    DNLM/DLC
    for Library of Congress   93-50880
                                                                    CIP

Foreword

As a medical student or new house officer enters a busy Labor and Delivery corridor, it is easy to become overwhelmed. A natural reaction is to turn to currently available textbooks in order to increase one's knowledge and thereby more effectively cope with patient problems. However, most texts address the principles of clinical medicine without emphasizing the relevant, practical application. Further, commonly encountered problems are often buried among the obscure and trivial, serving to confuse rather than to elucidate.

This unique handbook promises to help the obstetrics clerk survive and enjoy his or her obstetrical experience. First, it is more easily readable than most medical texts and can be entirely digested in about 3 hours. Second, it is designed to emphasize the clinical circumstances faced during the first obstetrics rotation, leaving one to turn to traditional texts for discussion of principles and pathophysiology. Third, it includes an easy approach to situations that are often assumed to be mundane but are described poorly or not at all in other texts. Examples are techniques for obtaining fetal scalp pH, placing a fetal scalp electrode or intrauterine pressure catheter, and performing a circumcision. The approach to obtaining a surgical consent and the proper manner of dictating a concise operative report are clearly detailed. Fourth, this text is cleverly organized by hospital geography rather than by disease and thereby introduces young physicians to problems that they will face in a given location.

This is not intended to be a comprehensive treatise on normal or complicated obstetrics. Rather, it is an attempt to facilitate the transition from being a student to being a clinician. As one who has been actively involved in medical student and resident education for the last 14 years, I applaud this novel endeavor as a valuable, efficient teaching aid.

Michael L. Socol, MD
Associate Professor and Head
Section of Maternal-Fetal Medicine
Department of Obstetrics and Gynecology
Northwestern University Medical School
Chicago, Illinois

Preface

When a resident rotates through obstetrics for the first time, he or she will probably seek help from the many texts available. Unfortunately, this wealth of information will be largely irrelevant to the task of just getting through the day at the outset of the obstetrics rotation. Why isn't more effective and immediate help given to the resident who seems to have no escape from psychological pressure? The answer is that few medical educators make a clear distinction between information necessary to know in the first month of a particular rotation and those facts important for specialty certification. This contributes to the "hazing" that young physicians experience as they begin a new rotation.

The standard manuals and texts often fall short of providing specific information most urgently needed. How often should progress notes be written on laboring patients? What should I do to prepare the patient for cesarean section? What if a mother suddenly delivers in the labor room and I am the only physician available?

I wrote *Obstetrical Pearls* when I was a senior obstetrics resident responsible for overseeing labor and delivery. Among my responsibilities at that time was to be the primary teacher for medical students, ER residents rotating for 2 months through ob-gyn, and first and second-year obstetrical residents. I found that everyone asked the same questions and that there was no single, easy-to-master source of information that could help them.

The purpose of this text is to give residents and medical students in an obstetrics rotation precise instructions about what to do and write in specific clinical situations. Clearly, some of the recommendations in this book are controversial. The value of this information is that it provides one approach to commonly encountered problems so that the inexperienced physician will have some guide when help is not readily available. Best of all, the book can be read completely in about 3 hours the night before the obstetrics rotation.

The book has been organized around the three clinical settings encountered as an obstetrical resident: the obstetrical clinic for antepartum care, labor and delivery, and the postpartum floor. In many institutions, residents will move from one area to another several times in the course of a day. A fourth part includes a variety of relatively uncommon conditions in which junior residents may occasionally become involved.

It has been 4 years since the first edition of *Obstetrical Pearls* has appeared. The enthusiastic response it has received has far exceeded my expectations. The book has been translated into Spanish, and an Asian company has just bought the rights to translate it into Japanese. It is available in Mexico, India, Portugal, and Singapore. In view of the book's success, the publisher and I have produced this second edition to keep the book current. Although 4 years may not seem to be a long time, new antibiotics are being used, and recommendations for specific conditions have changed.

Obstetrical Pearls may not help the resident or student score high marks in knowledge tests, and it is not a substitute for reading and mastering the more extensive texts on obstetrics. Only the more common clinical situations are addressed here. Guidelines are set forth that are meant to be generalizations and naturally do not apply in every situation and under every circumstance. Yet, this information should help the uninitiated deal successfully with the obstetrics environment when thrust into it for the first time.

MDB

Contents

1
PART

Prenatal Care

1

The Initial Assessment

INITIAL HISTORY

The initial history and physical for obstetrics is similar to that in other rotations. Although it shares features of the labor and delivery history and physical described in a later section, the emphasis is different. Most clinics use a standardized form that is self-explanatory. If not, the history portion can follow the format below.

History of Present Illness

This part of the initial history should focus particularly on prior types of contraception, menstrual history, first positive pregnancy test, and symptoms of pregnancy.

A source of constant confusion is that of gravidity and parity. Gravidity refers to the total number of pregnancies, including the present one. Multiple gestations are counted as only one pregnancy. Parity describes pregnancy outcome. One method to record parity is to use the T-P-A-L system in which "T" stands for term, "P" indicates preterm deliveries, "A" refers to abortions (whether elective or spontaneous), and "L" is the number of offspring currently alive. "Full-term" in this case means that the fetus was delivered at 37 completed weeks or beyond. In other words, "term" defines a period from 14 days before the due date to 14 days after the due date. An abortion is the intended or unintended delivery of the pregnancy before the fetus completed 20 weeks or achieved 500 g. Premature is that time period after 20 weeks and before term.

Past Medical History

Prior abdominal surgery, major medical conditions, and previous pregnancy outcomes are of special interest.

Family History

Predispositions for illness in the mother, such as heart disease or diabetes, are important and include genetic issues for the fetus. This refers to birth defects in the families of either parent-to-be as well as their ethnic backgrounds.

Social History

Substance abuse is of supreme interest here because smoking, alcohol, and drugs can all cause bad outcomes that are presumably preventable. When asking about drug use, phrase the question, "Do you use any recreational drugs such as marijuana or cocaine?" The response is bound to be different than if you say, "You do not use any illegal drugs, do you?" The prospective mother's economic circumstances and living conditions are also relevant.

Review of Systems

Inquire about symptoms characteristic of pregnancy: heartburn, gas, constipation, nausea, breast tenderness, and the like.

INITIAL PHYSICAL EXAM

The physical exam should include all major body systems, with particular emphasis on the abdomen and pelvis. Scars, presence of heart tones, and uterine size should be included in the abdominal exam. For the pelvic exam, cervical dilatation and effacement as well as uterine size

Figure 1–1. The maternal pelvis. (Adapted from Bonica, JJ: Principles and Practice of Obstetric Analgesia and Anesthesia. FA Davis, Philadelphia, 1967, p 851, with permission.)

are of interest. Pelvimetry, or estimation of the size of the bony pelvis, is particularly difficult for beginners, but an effort can be made to note some of the most obvious landmarks, which are indicated below and in Figure 1–1.

Conjugate Diameter

This is defined as the distance from the lower aspect of pubic symphysis to the sacral promontory. To measure this, simply palpate as far upward and backward as possible. Unless you have long fingers, you often will not be able to feel the sacral promontory. In this event, simply note that the "CD" is greater than the measured length of your outstretched fingers.

Sacrum

Is it hollow or flat? This is a subjective assessment.

Coccyx

Is it anterior or posterior? Again, a matter of judgment.

Ischial Spines

These are the bony protuberances at 4:00 and 8:00, 2 inches or so into the vaginal canal along the vaginal sidewalls. Are they prominent?

Transverse Diameter

This is the distance between the ischial tuberosities and can best be examined with the patient flat with her legs adducted and dorsiflexed (the position for a routine pelvic exam). They are the broad bony prominences that are palpable on the medial aspect of the buttocks, inferior to the anus.

Pubic Arch Angle

This can be estimated by sweeping two fingers under the pubic arch. Women commonly have an arch angle of 110° or greater.

Pelvimetry is of limited importance in the prenatal evaluation because in most cases, cephalopelvic disproportion (fetus too large for the pelvis) is empirically determined by observing the course of labor.

DATING THE PREGNANCY

This is one of the most important tasks in prenatal care.

Last Menstrual Period

It is often stated that 40% of women do not accurately recall their last menstrual period (LMP). The following facts need to be stated in the chart at the first visit:

1. First day of last menstrual period and whether or not it was normal.
2. The length and variability of the patient's menstrual cycles (when not on oral contraceptives).
3. Presence or absence of pill use or breastfeeding within 6 months prior to conception. These factors can result in delayed ovulation for several subsequent cycles.

First Fetal Movement (Quickening)

Primigravidas generally feel the first fetal movement at 18 to 20 weeks, whereas women with their second pregnancy and beyond feel the fetus move 2 weeks earlier.

Fetal Heartbeat

The heart can be heard with the fetoscope as early as 17 weeks and usually by 20 weeks. The heartbeat can usually be heard with a Doppler instrument by 12 weeks. From 16 weeks and beyond it is important to document how the heart tones were detected. In this time period, one should always listen with the fetoscope, as the first date on which the heartbeat can be heard with this instrument can help confirm the due date. In the first two trimesters, the fetal heartbeat is most commonly heard close to the midline.

Fundal Height

Measure from the top of the symphysis pubis.

12 weeks: Palpable abdominally just at the symphysis pubis.
16 weeks: Palpable midway between the symphysis and the umbilicus.
20 weeks: Palpable at the umbilicus.
20 to 32 weeks: Height in centimeters above symphysis parallels gestational age in weeks.

While the above serves as a rule of thumb, interobserver and intraobserver variability is very high. Assuming that one ultrasound has been previously done to confirm the due date, additional scans based on discrepancies in the physical exam are warranted only in the more extreme cases.

Ultrasound

1. First trimester: Crown-rump length predicts the estimated date of confinement (EDC, or due date) to within 7 to 10 days.
2. Second trimester: Biparietal diameter (BPD) or femur length predicts EDC to within 7 to 10 days.
3. Third trimester: Scans postponed to this time period are not very helpful in predicting the EDC and are accurate only to within 3 weeks either way.

As a rule, when an early ultrasound prediction disagrees with an EDC assigned by the LMP by more than 1 week, the ultrasound dates are assigned. If the scan and the LMP agree to within a week, the EDC based on the LMP is used. This may not always be straightforward because femur length may or may not agree with the estimated gestational age based on the biparietal diameter. Ultrasound is not the last word on dating a pregnancy and must be used in combination with the above observations.

If there is any question concerning the due date assigned on the basis of LMP, an ultrasound should be considered to help clarify the issue. Most patients presenting after 18 weeks should probably be scanned at least once. They should also be scanned if there is a large discrepancy between dates and size or if the uterus does not seem to be growing on several successive visits.

REFERRAL TO HIGH-RISK CLINIC

Many residency programs have more than one obstetrical clinic or make consultation available for so called high-risk patients. The following are examples of problems that warrant referral to the high-risk clinic or consultation (when available) for follow-up on future visits:

1. History of preterm delivery (<36 weeks or weight <5 pounds, 8 ounces).
2. Prior intrauterine fetal demise (IUFD)—stillbirth.
3. Pregnancy loss between 14 and 20 weeks (suggestive of incompetent cervix).
4. Multiple gestation.
5. Third trimester bleeding or the discovery of placenta previa or any of its variations after 26 to 28 weeks' gestation.
6. Isoimmunization.
7. Presence of serious systemic disease, e.g., diabetes, hypertension, asthma, renal or cardiac disease, etc.
8. History of deep venous thrombosis (not varicose veins) or pulmonary embolus.

2

CHAPTER

Routine Prenatal Visits

Patients are seen monthly until 28 weeks and then every 2 weeks. After 36 weeks, patients are seen weekly. The following items are checked with every prenatal visit.

WEIGHT

Ideally, a patient should gain about 25 to 35 pounds during her pregnancy—roughly $1/2$ pound per week for the first 28 weeks and 1 pound per week thereafter. Many gravidas will not stick closely to this pattern. Obese patients may gain substantially less. Mothers who are gaining too much weight should be encouraged to avoid snacks; watch their consumption of high-calorie fluids (soda pop, even juices and milk); and stick to three well-balanced meals per day. Weight gain of more than 5 pounds per week at the end of pregnancy may be a sign of preeclampsia, and the urine and blood pressure should be checked closely. Those with extremes of weight gain should have their eating habits reviewed and should be referred to a dietician if one is available. Weight loss that occurs over more than one visit is of particular concern.

Patients often ask about the safety of artificial sweeteners such as aspartame (NutraSweet). A modified amino acid, aspartame is not a known or suspected teratogen or mutagen, and it has been in the food supply for several decades. Even for mothers carrying a fetus with phenylketonuria, the additive is safe, as the mother's enzymes break it down; carriers of phenylketonuria are able to do so. In a real sense, aspartame is safer than sugar, since chronic exposure to large doses of sugar may lead to obesity and increased risk of Cesarean section and diabetes.

BLOOD PRESSURE

The maternal blood pressure tends to drop in the second trimester and rise in the third trimester.

Guidelines for Concern

1. Diastolic greater than 85
2. Systolic of 140 or greater
3. Mean arterial pressure of 105 or greater
      (systolic BP + 2 × diastolic BP)/3
4. Rise in systolic of 30
5. Rise in diastolic of 15

Work-up

1. Repeat blood pressure both sitting up and in lateral decubitus (upper arm).
2. 24-hour urine for total protein and creatinine clearance.
3. SMA-20. If in third trimester, also CBC with platelets to evaluate for preeclampsia.

4. Stat urinalysis if dipstick urine indicates more than 1+ protein on a voided specimen. A catheterized specimen should be obtained if patient has heavy vaginal discharge.

Follow-up

If elevated blood pressures are recorded at the time of the first visit in the first or early second trimester, they may indicate that the patient is a chronic hypertensive.

If these pressures are newly elevated and recorded in the late second trimester or third trimester, the patient may well have preeclampsia. An experienced resident should be notified, because the patient may need to be hospitalized for observation. At the very least, she should be rechecked in 2 to 3 days, and a nonstress test (NST—see Fetal Movement in Chapter 4) may be appropriate (depending on the gestational age and the absolute value of the blood pressure).

URINE DIPSTICK

Protein

A negative, trace, or 1+ reading requires no action. A 2+ or greater reading requires a clean-catch midstream urinalysis (hold for culture and sensitivity). If it is suggestive of a urinary tract infection, the patient may be treated presumptively. She should call 2 or 3 days later for the culture results. The blood pressure must be checked to be sure it is not elevated. Proteinuria can be a sign of preeclampsia if accompanied by elevated blood pressure.

Glucose

Although the threshold for glucosuria in pregnancy is reduced, in practice, glucose rarely is positive on the dipsticks. If 2+ glucose is found on a urine dipstick, it may be appropriate to perform the routine diabetes screen earlier than the usual 24 to 28 weeks (see Blood Sugar and Diabetes in Chapter 3). If a screen has already been done, and glucosuria is a repeated finding in the third trimester, there may be merit in rechecking the screening test or even obtaining a more definitive 3-hour glucose tolerance test.

FUNDAL HEIGHT AND FETAL HEARTBEAT

See Dating the Pregnancy in Chapter 1.

EDEMA

Seventy-five percent of pregnant women ultimately complain of edema. Thus, it is not a very useful screening sign or symptom for pre-eclampsia. Those with excessive or sudden swelling should, of course, have their blood pressure and urine protein checked, but usually the swelling is an isolated finding. A good clue to excessive swelling is a weight gain of 3 pounds or more in a week.

Sitting with legs up or lying on one's side will help isolated edema. To be effective, the patient has to rest for several hours when she would not otherwise. In practice, most patients prefer to tolerate moderate leg swelling rather than lie in bed for several hours during the middle of the day.

FETAL MOVEMENT

This should be noted on each visit. The first perception by the patient (quickening) should also be noted. Specific instructions for the third trimester are reviewed under Fetal Movement in Chapter 4.

3

CHAPTER

Prenatal Labs

BLOOD SUGAR AND DIABETES

Several hormones of pregnancy are insulin antagonists. Chief among them is human placental lactogen (HPL), which is secreted by the placenta in rough proportion to its weight. Thus, women who have normal glucose tolerances in early pregnancy may actually be diabetic later in the gestation. Prior to the introduction of insulin, 50% of diabetic mothers died, and the fetal outcome was worse. This disease is important because it is reasonably common (1% to 2% of pregnant mothers) and because we can have a significant impact on its outcome.

Risk Factors

The following features of a patient's initial assessment suggest that the patient is at higher than average risk for diabetes.

RF
for
DM

1. Prior stillbirth
2. Prior fetus weighing over 9 pounds
3. Strong family history of diabetes
4. Morbid obesity
5. Glucosuria

Screening Policy

1. All pregnancies should be screened between 24 and 28 weeks with a 1-hour postprandial glucose test. This is a blood draw 1 hour after the patient consumes a 50-g glucose load. Many institutions do this after an overnight fast, but others simply administer the glucose during the regular appointment anytime during the day.
2. Those with an abnormal 1-hour postprandial glucose should have the 3-hour glucose tolerance test as soon as possible. If this test is abnormal, the patient is referred immediately to the diabetic or high-risk clinic.
3. Patients at high risk for gestational diabetes by history might benefit from a glucose screen at presentation or a second screening test at 32 weeks.

The 1-Hour Postprandial Glucose

The patient can be given a 50-g oral glucose load after fasting for 8 hours and have her glucose checked 1 hour later. A fasting (or pretest) glucose is not measured with this screen. The cut-off value varies among institutions, but it is usually considered abnormal if it is higher than 135 or 140 (mg/100 mL). About 15% of the population will have an abnormal 1-hour test with this cut-off.

The 3-Hour Glucose Tolerance Test

The patient is to have 100-g carbohydrate intake for 3 days prior to the test. The test requires administration of a 100-g glucose load and then checking the plasma glucose at fasting, 1 hour, 2 hours, and 3 hours. The upper limit of normal for each of the values (plasma—in mg/100 mL) is:

Fasting: 105
1 Hour: 190
2 Hours: 165
3 Hours: 145

The test is abnormal if two or more values exceed the upper limit of normal.

Classifying Diabetes

A gestational diabetic is one whose 3-hour glucose tolerance test is abnormal and who was not known to be diabetic prior to the pregnancy. This definition is known to encompass a very heterogeneous group and may include those who should have been on insulin before the pregnancy. (Most women are screened for the first time during pregnancy.) One commonly used classification scheme for describing diabetes in pregnant women (based on the White system) is described below.

Class A-1: Fasting glucose <105.
Class A-2: Fasting glucose ≥105—these patients are usually started on insulin.
Class B-1: Fasting glucose ≥130.
Class B-2: Adult onset (type II) diabetics (on insulin prior to pregnancy).
Class C: Diabetes onset between ages 10 and 19.
Class D: Diabetes of more than 20 years' duration or beginning before age 10.
Class F: Concomitant nephropathy.
Class R: Malignant retinopathy.

Diabetes of any degree establishes a pregnancy as "high risk" and requires consultation of more senior residents or faculty members.

Problems Faced by Pregnant Diabetics

There are three special types of difficulties faced by diabetics during pregnancy. The risk of congenital malformation, particularly in the heart and nervous system, is greatly increased (especially in those with abnormal glucose tolerance in the first trimester). Generally, these patients have a twofold to fourfold increase in risk, which tends to be higher in those under poor control. The risk of stillbirth is also significantly increased. Finally, macrosomia, in which the fetus attains an excessive size, is of concern as this predisposes to shoulder dystocia and cephalopelvic disproportion. For these reasons, diabetic patients should have nonstress tests (NSTs—see Fetal Movement in Chapter 4) performed weekly beginning at 30 to 32 weeks, and frequent ultrasounds to look for malformations and predict macrosomia. An experienced obstetrician should be present at the delivery of a diabetic as shoulder dystocia can be a serious problem.

Gestational diabetics who are not on insulin postpartum may require insulin if placed on oral contraceptives. Thus, the pill is relatively contraindicated for these patients. If these patients are given oral contraceptives, their glucose tolerance needs to be watched carefully.

Approximately half of gestational diabetics will have abnormal glucose tolerance later in life.

HEMATOCRIT

All patients should be given vitamins and iron at the initial prenatal visit. Hematocrits are routinely rechecked early in the third trimester. For women with values under 30, the importance of iron should be stressed, and supplemental iron may need to be increased. A complete blood count with platelets and a ferritin should be performed. Subsequent work-up depends on these initial findings and the response to iron. A purely iron-deficiency anemia will usually respond to iron supplementation within 2 weeks.

Rh AND ANTIBODY SCREEN

Rh-negative mothers receive a passive immunization at 28 weeks to prevent hemolytic disease of the newborn. Without the vaccine before and after birth, Rh-negative mothers may develop antibodies to the Rh antigen if their fetus is Rh positive. In future pregnancies, these IgG antibodies can cross the placenta and destroy Rh-positive fetal red blood cells. This may lead to severe anemia and death for subsequent Rh-positive fetuses. While most maternal Rh immunization takes place at the time of birth with the entrance of fetal red blood cells into the bloodstream, a small percentage of pregnant women will be exposed to fetal red blood cells before labor and thus become immunized.

The immunization consists of an injection at 28 weeks with IgG antibody to the Rh antigen. One common brand name of this vaccine is RhoGAM. If an antibody screen is done within weeks (or even 2 to 3 months) after this injection, it may be positive. These mothers also must receive RhoGAM for amniocentesis or any other event that places them at increased risk for fetal-maternal transfusion (such as an abortion). The mothers also receive RhoGAM in the first three days postpartum if their child is indeed Rh-positive. It must be remembered that an antibody screen must always be checked prior to giving

RhoGAM at any time to be sure that Rh sensitization has not already taken place.

All positive antibody screens require consultation.

RUBELLA TITER

Most cases of rubella (German mcaslcs) are subclinical, so the history is completely unreliable. The rubella virus is a teratogen capable of causing cardiac defects, cataracts, and deafness in the fetus. Nonimmune women should be vaccinated postpartum as all vaccines use an attenuated live strain of virus and are theoretically teratogenic in and of themselves, although this has not been the case in actual practice. All patients are routinely screened for immunity, and those with borderline values should have the test repeated to be sure that they do not have a current infection.

Those who are vaccinated should avoid pregnancy for 3 months. They are not contagious. The vaccination does not prohibit breast-feeding.

PAP SMEAR

Pap smear abnormalities can be of two types: those suggesting the presence of an infectious disease and those read out as dysplasia. Infectious diseases identified on a Pap smear (yeast, trichomonas, etc.) do not need to be treated if the patient is asymptomatic.

Pap smears that are frankly abnormal are classified as a low- or high-grade "squamous intraepithelial lesion." The low-grade lesions may be categorized as condyloma and mild dysplasia, and the high-grade lesions as moderate or severe dysplasia (including carcinoma in situ). With the high-grade lesions, an examination with a colposcope (a type of magnifying glass) and directed biopsies of the cervix are performed in order to exclude malignancy and determine frequency of follow-up. The proper follow-up of low-grade lesions is controversial, however, particularly during pregnancy. An alternative to colposcopy and biopsy may be simply follow-up Pap smears at intervals of 3 to 6 months, although the recommendation has to be individualized according to the patient's medical history and likelihood of compliance.

Treatment, such as freezing or lasering of the cervix, is usually postponed to the postpartum period as long as the lesion is not invasive cancer.

The Pap smear can occasionally be normal in the presence of cancer. Cervices that appear to be very abnormal or that have fungating, indurated regions should be brought to the attention of an experienced examiner. More often than not, the cervix is actually normal, but keep in mind that a normal Pap smear does not absolutely exclude cancer.

MATERNAL SERUM ALPHA-FETOPROTEIN

Recently, a maternal blood test has become available to screen for fetuses with neural tube defects. This group of congenital anomalies occurs at the rate of roughly 1 in 1000 pregnancies (5 in 1000 in the British isles) and includes a variety of conditions such as spina bifida and anencephaly (fetus missing cerebral cortex). High levels of a specific protein, alpha-fetoprotein (AFP), in the maternal bloodstream may suggest an afflicted fetus.

In the past few years, the test's predictive value has been improved by adding a concomitant assay for HCG, estradiol, or both. This improved test is also known as the AFP plus test or the "triple screen." The addition of a second or even third protein assay makes interpretation of the test significantly more complicated. In many labs, a narrative report accompanies the interpretation. In the case of abnormal values, the lab will typically recommend a specific follow-up (i.e., a repeat test, ultrasound, or amniocentesis).

When available, the test is done between 15 and 20 weeks. Abnormal values are to be called to the attention of an experienced resident. (Most institutions have a standard protocol about the follow-up of these tests.) With most screening procedures, about 30 to 50 mothers out of 1000 will have an initial abnormal AFP (against a background incidence of 1 to 2:1,000 with an actual defect). Those morally opposed to abortion may decline this test. Abnormally high AFP levels can occur from incorrect gestational age assignment, twins, and fetal demise.

Women with one abnormal test (generally 2.5 multiples of the median or higher) should have an ultrasound to confirm the gestational age and rule out twins. If the scan disagrees by 2 weeks or more with the age assigned by the last menstrual period, the gestational age is changed and the result reinterpreted. If the value remains abnormal, the patient undergoes a combination of genetic counseling and then amniocentesis and an ultrasound to look for anomalies (if she agrees). Unusually low values (0.5 multiples of the median or less) may predict an increased risk of chromosomal abnormalities (such as Down's syndrome) and should be treated in the same way.

The protocol for following up an abnormal initial test varies among institutions. Whatever method is used, it is important to recognize that the normal range is highly dependent on gestational age and that unusually high or low levels of AFP need to be pursued.

HEMOGLOBIN ELECTROPHORESIS

Those who are homozygous for variant hemoglobins are followed in a high-risk clinic. Those with sickle cell trait need to be counseled about the possibility of testing the fetus for sickle cell disease should the father also have the trait (he must be brought in and tested). In these cases, the fetal genotype should be determined before 20 weeks through amniocentesis or chorionic villus sampling. These patients also need urine cultures checked once a month, as they are predisposed to urinary tract infections. Other hemoglobin electrophoresis abnormalities require consultation.

ULTRASOUND

The availability of ultrasound examination and protocols for routine scanning vary greatly among institutions. Nevertheless, once an ultrasound is obtained, the following is a partial list of findings that require consultation:

1. High risk for intrauterine growth retardation (IUGR).
2. Macrosomia (unusually large fetus).
3. Oligohydramnios (abnormally low volume of amniotic fluid).
4. Hydramnios (abnormally high volume of amniotic fluid).
5. Breech presentation or transverse lie after 35 weeks (no need for action before this time).

6. Placenta previa (after 28 weeks—sooner if bleeding).

GENETIC TESTING

Two prenatal tests are available that can identify fetuses with chromosome errors and some specific genetic anomalies: amniocentesis and chorionic villus sampling (CVS). The field is advancing so rapidly that any statements committed to print quickly become obsolete. Even so, a few brief principles are worth reviewing.

Amniocentesis

The gold standard of genetic testing, amniocentesis has traditionally been done from 14 to 18 weeks—a time when enough fluid has accumulated to make the test easy to perform but early enough so that if the results are abnormal, the patient can undergo a pregnancy termination. The most common reason for doing the test is to study the fetal chromosomes.

While there are several different classes of congenital anomalies, chromosome errors are the only type of defect to increase in frequency with advancing maternal age. Since these defects are often severe or even lethal (one example is Down's syndrome), it has become common practice to offer prenatal diagnosis for chromosome errors to women who will be 35 years old or older at the time of delivery. This is the first age at which the probability of finding a chromosome error (roughly 1 in 170) exceeds the risk of spontaneous abortion from the procedure itself (1 in 200). The technique relies on the fact that fetal cells shed into the amniotic fluid are still viable and can be cultured to build up enough volume of cells for analysis. Because the cells have to multiply before testing can be performed, it usually takes 3 to 4 weeks to have a karyotype (chromosome count) from the amniotic fluid.

With the advances in biotechnology, an ever-lengthening list of specific genetic errors can also be identified. Examples include Tay-Sachs disease and, recently, sickle cell anemia. However, amniocentesis is not appropriate for all mothers, and not all tests available can be performed on each fluid sample. Rather, the initial history is used to identify people at increased risk for one or more genetic problems. The most obvious risk is mothers who will be age 35 or older at the time of delivery, but certain ethnic groups might also benefit from genetic screening and, occasionally, amniocentesis. For example, if both members of a Jewish couple are carrying the Tay-Sachs gene, a genetic amniocentesis can prenatally identify those 25% of babies who will have the fatal homozygous disease.

Chorionic Villus Sampling

CVS is a relatively new technique that involves aspirating a very small portion of the placenta at 9 to 11 weeks. The placenta has the fetal karyotype rather than the maternal one. The actual aspiration is performed with ultrasound guidance and can be done either transvaginally or transabdominally. CVS can be done 6 to 8 weeks earlier than amniocentesis, and the results can usually be obtained with a week, since a greater number of fetal cells are obtained from the outset with this technique. CVS can be used both for karyotypes and identifying specific genetic errors, but it cannot yet be used to screen for neural tube defects because this requires measurement of amniotic fluid AFP. Rarely, a patient who undergoes CVS will have an elevated serum AFP and require amniocentesis.

The compelling advantage of CVS is that results can be obtained in the first trimester rather than the second trimester as with amniocentesis. This is of great practical importance for those who wish to terminate an abnormal pregnancy. The disadvantage of CVS is its slightly higher loss rate (on the order of 1 to 2 per 200) when compared with the 1 per 200 of amniocentesis.) It is helpful to realize that most pregnancy losses after either procedure would have occurred anyway. Specifically, 6 in 200 pregnancies viable at 16 weeks are subsequently lost. This number rises only to 7 in 200 after amniocentesis.

4

CHAPTER

Common Concerns and Problems of Pregnant Women

FETAL MOVEMENT

If a patient complains of decreased fetal movement after 28 weeks, she needs a nonstress test (NST) that day. An NST should not be ordered weekly thereafter for this nonrecurring problem.

The NST consists of electronically monitoring and recording the fetal pulse rate for a minimum of 20 minutes. A "reactive" NST is one that is reassuring about fetal well-being. While the definition of "reactive" varies among institutions, a common one is a pulse pattern with two or more accelerations lasting for at least 15 seconds within a 20-minute period with the peak of the acceleration being 15 bpm above the baseline fetal heart rate (FHR). The interpretation of FHR tracings is described in greater detail in Fetal Monitoring in Chapter 6.

With regard to monitoring fetal movement in general, there are a variety of different protocols for instructing patients. An example of one such guideline is as follows:

1. Upon awakening, begin counting your baby's movements.
2. A kick, punch, or roll each counts as one movement. If the baby kicks and then rolls, this should be counted as two movements.
3. Stop counting for the day when you reach 10. The baby is fine.
4. If you don't reach 10 by 5 PM, call your doctor. You will need to come in for an NST (the nurse will place a "microphone" on your abdomen for half an hour to hear the baby's pulse). Most babies are just fine.

The key principle is that any large change in the fetal daily activity requires follow-up. The stillbirth rate has been shown to decrease significantly among mothers who monitor their baby's movements daily.

VAGINAL INFECTIONS

Vaginal infections are treated because they cause symptoms and discomfort—not because they threaten the pregnancy or the health of the mother. Asymptomatic patients do not need treatment—particularly in the first trimester.

Monistat 7 vaginal suppositories may be used at any time during pregnancy, although preferably after the first trimester. Metronidazole should probably not be used in the first trimester and early second trimester since there is some concern that it may be a potential teratogen.

URINARY TRACT INFECTIONS

Treat as you would normally. Always check a culture following treatment. Never prescribe tetracycline during pregnancy and avoid, if possible, giving sulfa or nitrofurantoin after 36 weeks. Tetracycline administered during pregnancy can cause permanent discoloration of the offspring's teeth. Sulfa drugs administered close to the time of delivery can presumably displace bilirubin from its carrier molecules and theoretically can predispose to toxicity. Nitrofurantoin might exacerbate hemolytic anemias resulting from a specific enzyme deficiency, G-6-PD.

SEX

There are no restrictions placed on sex for the pregnant woman without specific medical or obstetrical problems. Air emboli resulting in maternal death have been reported in the medical literature from blowing air under pressure into the vagina during oral sex.

ABDOMINAL PAIN

Most pregnant women eventually complain of lower abdominal discomfort or pain. Sometimes this may actually be Braxton Hicks contractions, but often it is hard to find a specific cause. Occasionally, patients will be tender along the lateral aspects of the uterus. This condition is commonly referred to as "round ligament pain" since the pain corresponds roughly to the location of the round ligament, although the physiology behind the pain is poorly delineated. Mild abdominal aches and pains can be treated with a heating pad and Tylenol.

LEG CRAMPS

Many pregnant women experience painful leg cramping, particularly at night. The cause of these cramps is unknown. While uncomfortable, most patients are satisfied with reassurance that this is a normal discomfort of pregnancy. For those with particularly bad symptoms, supplemental calcium can be tried (although the evidence that this is of benefit is skimpy at best). Physical examination should be performed at some point, however, to rule out deep venous thrombosis. If the physical exam is suspicious (such as demonstrating asymmetric swelling, localized tenderness, cords, or erythema), duplex imaging should be ordered, as examination by itself is notoriously unreliable. Duplex imaging consists of a real-time ultrasound study of the venous circulation between the knee and the groin. Deep venous thromboses can actually be visualized with this technique.

$$\frac{2}{\text{PART}}$$

The Labor and Delivery Suite

5

CHAPTER

Initial Patient Evaluation

TRIAGE

The labor and delivery area is not used solely to take care of laboring patients at term. It also serves as a sort of emergency room for pregnant women who are not in labor. With its fetal heart rate monitors and heavy staffing of nurses, this ward is well suited for rapid evaluation of pregnant women and intervention, if necessary. When a patient presents to labor and delivery, her disposition depends on two things: (1) estimated gestational age (EGA) and (2) presenting complaint.

Gestational Age

If the estimated gestational age is equal to or greater than 36 weeks, an intern or junior resident can evaluate the patient. If less than 36 weeks, however, consultation should be obtained.

Presenting Complaint in Term Patient

Patients at term usually come to labor and delivery for one of two reasons: *contractions* or *ruptured membranes*. Obviously, those with a question of ruptured membranes but who are not contracting do not need to be seen as quickly as those with strong contractions.

ADMITTING WORK-UP

Requirements for this document vary among institutions. The history and physical outlined below are examples of what information is considered relevant in the work-up. In principle, a complete medical history is obtained at the first prenatal visit so that this history should not contain many surprises. It is acceptable to obtain most of the history from the prenatal record, although the important points should be double-checked with the patient.

For women in advanced labor who are in much pain, some of the information may be skipped. As an example, if someone is barely able to talk and already 5 cm dilated, it does not seem worthwhile to zealously pursue the accuracy of due date by obtaining a rigorous menstrual history. Also, many hospitals have abbreviated forms that make the admission work-up easier. The example below is rather detailed, and both time and the patient's discomfort may not permit a perfect document on every occasion.

HISTORY

Chief Complaint

Contractions and/or spontaneous rupture of membranes (SROM).

History of Present Illness

Ms. _____ is a (age), (race), G_____ P (Term-Preterm-Abortion-Living), LMP _____ , EDC _____ [by dates, exam, ultrasound (include those that are appropriate)] who presents to labor and delivery at ____ weeks complaining of _____ . The second sentence summarizes the membrane status and contraction pattern (always indicate the time of ruptured membranes). She has gained ____ pounds during an uncomplicated pregnancy (OR a pregnancy complicated by. . .).

Prenatal Labs

Rubella titer: (>1.0 or >1:8 shows immunity)
Blood type and Rh
Antibody screen
Other relevant positives or negatives
Ultrasound findings (if obtained)

Past Medical History

Hospitalizations, surgery, accidents
Medications
Allergies
Menstrual history: It is important to document whether regular or not when there is a question about the gestational age. Last oral contraceptive use, if relevant. Pill use within 3 to 6 months of the last menstrual period can delay ovulation and throw off dates.

Past Obstetrical History

Include maternal age plus gestational age, sex, weight, and route of delivery for each birth along with complications. This can often be copied from the prenatal record without troubling the laboring mother.

Social History

Smoking, alcohol, illicit drug use, who is in the household, and occupation.

Family History

Be brief, defer if pressed for time. Include only relevant details (diabetes, hypertension, history of twinning, etc.). Again, this can usually be obtained from the prenatal record.

Review of Systems

Only relevant positives.

EXAM (EXAMPLE)

Vitals
Pupils: equal and reactive to light accommodation
Throat: without erythema
Neck: without adenopathy, thyromegaly
Lungs: clear
Heart: RRR; S_1, S_2 with I/VI systolic murmur along the left sternal border
Back: without costovertebral angle tenderness
Abdomen:
     Fundal height (FH) = _____ cm.
     Estimated fetal weight (EFW) = _____.
     Fetal heart tones (FHTs) = _____.
     Contractions every _____ minutes (by palpation or monitor—indicate which).

Draw a picture of the fetus, indicating head and back location. Be circumspect before drawing anything other than vertex. Put an "X" in the location of the fetal heart tones. Be sure to note the presence of any abdominal scars.

Pelvic:

Dilatation: Between closed and 10 cm (also known as complete).

Effacement: The normal cervix is 2 to 3 cm long. Thickness is expressed as %. A completely thinned out cervix is 100% effaced.

Station: Distance in cm between the lowest bony portion of the fetus and the maternal ischial spines. Generally a number between −3 (above the spines) and +3 (below the spines).

Presenting part: If anything other than vertex is suspected, consultation should be obtained.

Note: When the cervix is dilated enough, usually by 5 cm, it should be possible to feel the sutures and thus also indicate position (orientation of the presenting part).

Status of membranes: Either intact or ruptured. There are three common methods of determining that membranes are ruptured: (1) fluid gushing from vagina (indicate whether clear or meconium-stained): (2) nitrazine positive (amniotic fluid has a pH between 7.1 and 7.4) while 90% of women will have acidic urine (thus allowing nitrazine to help distinguish between them): and (3) presence of ferning. Occasionally, cervical mucus can fern, so it is important to collect fluid from the posterior vault rather than the cervix itself.

Lower extremities

Deep tendon reflexes (DTRs):

Clonus

Edema

Calf tenderness

Note: Patients in labor normally have slightly increased DTRs, and up to two beats of clonus is considered normal. Up to 75% of pregnant women develop ankle edema at some point.

Impression

Patient is a _____ year old, (race), G _____ P _____ female at _____ weeks who presents to labor and delivery . . .

Plan

Admit. Monitor. Anticipate spontaneous vaginal birth. . . . It is helpful to check with the decision maker (attending or experienced resident) before committing a plan to paper if there is question about the proper course of action.

TIPS ON DOING THE WORK-UP

The key to being proficient in labor and delivery is to focus on brevity, completeness, and speed in performing admitting histories and physicals. Ideally, nothing should be written that is not immediately relevant, but nothing important should be left out. This is a skill that can only be obtained through experience.

Most of the history can be obtained from the nurse's admitting notes and the prenatal. Obtaining the information this way is faster and spares the patient repetitive questioning at a time when she is in pain. It is also faster to record the history directly on paper as it is being obtained. Leave a few blank lines for filling in all the specifics of the history of present illness that can be done after you see the patient. On the physical exam, the two most important aspects that require completeness are the abdominal and pelvic exams.

In this sample history and physical, I have omitted items that I consider to be unnecessary. Specifically, the breast exam on a patient in labor is often unreliable. Laboriously recording all of the prenatal labs such as the serology and Pap smear also seems to be a fruitless waste of time. All of these items are addressed in advance of labor or in the postpartum period and are rarely relevant to the management of labor. Admittedly, my opinions about what is important and unimportant in the work-up are not universally shared. In the absence of an explicit policy, the guidelines offered here are a good starting point.

NOTIFICATION OF THE APPROPRIATE PHYSICIAN OF THE PATIENT'S VISIT TO LABOR AND DELIVERY

This procedure varies in institutions. In most cases, private obstetricians like to be called (day or night) with the initial evaluation of their patient. They also usually like to be notified prior to administering any pain medication to their patients. They need to be kept up to date on the progress of labor so that they can have time to get to the hospital for the delivery. Again, policies about consultation with the private physicians vary among hospitals and individual attendings. Overconsultation is not irresponsible or a sign of poor judgment. Lack of authorization for specific actions, however, is to be avoided. Nurses can be a good source of practical advice. When in doubt, call.

6

CHAPTER

Care of the Laboring Patient

NORMAL AND ABNORMAL PROGRESS IN LABOR

In predicting the length of labor, it is important to keep in mind some basic definitions and concepts. First, obstetrical labor is not merely the occurrence of contractions but rather the progressive effacement and dilatation of the cervix in the presence of regular contractions. <u>Contractions without at least some initial dilatation is not labor</u>. The diagnosis of labor is necessarily a retrospective one as it is not always easy to distinguish between those having contractions and those having contractions that will lead to dilatation.

Most of the information about the length of "normal" labors and, indeed, the so-called labor curve itself comes from investigations conducted by Emanuel Friedman. Thus the frequent references to the "Friedman curve" in the labor suite. A more thorough discussion of labor can be found in Friedman's book, *Labor: Clinical Evaluation and Management.*

Important Definitions

First Stage. This begins with cervical efface-ment and dilatation and ends with complete dilatation.

The first stage is further divided into a *latent phase* and an *active phase*. The <u>latent phase</u> begins with cervical change in the presence of regular contractions. The <u>active phase</u> that follows begins with an increasing rate of cervical dilatation. As with labor itself, these divisions of the first stage are retrospective diagnoses. In most women, the latent phase ends and the active phase begins at 4 cm dilatation.

Second Stage. Begins with complete dilatation and ends with the birth of the baby. Mothers push during this stage.

Third Stage. Ends with the delivery of the placenta.

Orientation of Fetus with Descent

At term, 96% to 97% of fetuses present head first. Of those in cephalic presentation, 95% emerge as occiput anterior. That is, the back of the fetal head is rotated anteriorly with respect to the maternal pelvis. Occiput anterior fetuses emerge with their face toward the mother's rectum. Occiput posterior babies are born facing the symphysis pubis and are also known as "sunny-side up" babies. Labor, par-ticularly the second stage, often can take longer with such "posterior" babies. There is a widespread belief that "back labor," in which the center of pain is located in the lower back, is more frequent with occiput posterior fetuses, although the evidence for this is largely anecdotal.

As labor progresses, a change in the orientation

of the sutures can often be noted. With descent, the fetus will change from transverse (facing one maternal hip or the other) to anterior (facing the buttocks).

Limits of Normal

The following limits are published by Friedman. It is critical to realize that these numbers are *not* averages but limits of normal. That is, 95% of laboring women will accomplish a given portion of labor within the listed time interval.

First Labors

First stage:
    Latent phase—20.1 h (mean 6.4 h)
    Active phase—11.7 h (mean 4.6 h)
      Maximum dilatation >1.2 cm/h
        (mean 3 cm/h)
      Maximum descent >1 cm/h
        (mean 3.3 cm/h)
Second stage:
    2.9 h

Second Labors

First stage:
    Latent phase—13.6 h (mean 4.8 h)
    Active phase—5.2 h (mean 2.4 h)
      Maximum dilatation >1.5 cm/h
        (mean 5.7 cm/h)
      Maximum descent >2.1 cm/h
        (mean 6.6 cm/h)
Second stage:
    1.1 h

Of course, dilatation is not the only parameter to measure in labor. Complete effacement is usually accomplished by 4 to 5 cm of dilatation. More important, the presenting part must descend at some point, or the baby will not be born.

Women with their first labors will often have the presenting part engaged (at zero station) early in labor or before the onset of regular contractions. Women with subsequent labors will begin with the presenting part still high in the pelvis. In these women, it is not unusual for the head to be relatively high with complete dilatation.

Treatment of Abnormal Labor Patterns

Prolonged Latent Phase. Oxytocin infusion and narcotic sedation are both effective in ending an abnormally long latent phase, although oxytocin is somewhat faster. Amniotomy (artificial rupture of membranes) does not seem to be of benefit, although many believe that it is in spite of the data. Prolonged latent phase has not been associated with an increased incidence of subsequent labor abnormalities or a detrimental perinatal outcome.

Protracted Active Phase. The contractions may not be effective enough. Alternatively, the baby can be relatively large or poorly positioned.

Arrested Active Phase. There are basically only two reasons for a complete halt of progress in labor: poor contractions or cephalopelvic disproportion.

At this point, it is worth discussing "the three Ps." This concept seems to be universally taught to all medical students and has remained unchanged for at least 100 years. "The three Ps" refer to the powers, the passenger, and the pelvis. Unfortunately, this concept does not seem to have any empirical grounding and appears to be the cause of much confusion. After delivering 2000 babies, I make no claim to be able to distinguish between a big fetus versus a small maternal pelvis. The idea that somehow we can distinguish between the two has led to some very peculiar outcomes—including cesareans before the onset of labor because "the fetus is too big" or the "pelvis is too small." In practice, these clinical judgments cannot be made reliably without observing the progress in a labor with adequate contractions. Perhaps the three Ps should be replaced with "the two Ps"—the powers and the progress.

The frequency of contractions can be assessed by an external tocodynamometer, but the adequacy of contractions can be assessed only by palpation, the progress of labor, or with an intrauterine pressure catheter (IUPC, described later). The minimal strength of an effective contraction is thought to be in the range of 40 mm Hg. The normal resting tone for the uterus is under 20 mm Hg.

In most labors, contractions occur every 2 to 4 minutes. Oxytocin can be used if the contractions are not frequent or strong enough. On the other hand, contractions can occur too frequently and thereby compromise uteroplacental blood flow. This "tachysystole," or five or more contractions in 10 minutes, can be treated with hydration, lateral decubitus positioning of the patient, and oxygen.

If the contractions have proved to be adequate by an IUPC and no descent or dilatation has been made over 2 hours, the diagnosis of cephalopelvic disproportion (CPD) can be made. The treatment for CPD is cesarean section. There are several important caveats to bear in mind. First, cephalopelvic disproportion before 4 cm dilatation is unusual, and it is important to be sure that lack of expected progress is not merely due to the fact that the patient is in the latent phase of labor. Furthermore, the diagnosis of CPD is more reliably assigned if the presenting part is definitely "stuck." If descent or dilatation has occurred over 2 hours, the fetus may still be born vaginally.

The diagnosis of arrested active phase is not as easy to make in practice as it might sound. As the fetus descends, the head undergoes molding. In some cases, the head may actually be "stuck" but may undergo enough molding to give the false appearance of progress. Furthermore, caput (scalp edema) may develop and also give the illusion of progress. The presence of significant edema and molding on pelvic exam should increase the suspicion of possible CPD.

CPD is a diagnosis made on the empirical observation of labor. It cannot be reliably predicted from x-ray or ultrasound measurements of either the maternal pelvis or the fetus. The term has no universally accepted definition. Many obstetricians substitute the term "failure to progress," although this term also has no clear definition. Perhaps the best way to think of CPD is to view it as a reference to the fact that the fetal skeleton cannot pass through the maternal skeleton (in vertex presentation). This concept eliminates speculation about whether the fetus is too big or the pelvis too small, or whether the fetus is malrotated. If the fetus is occiput posterior or asynclitic (head tilted awkwardly in the sagittal plane), is the position the cause of the failed progress, or did the fetus end up in this position because it was the easiest fit in the first place? The answer is unknowable and academic. A fetus who is not born despite adequate contractions may be thought of as having CPD—its skeleton simply could not pass through the maternal skeleton.

Transfer of Patient to Delivery Room

In response to consumer demand, many hospitals have designed their rooms to be both a labor room and a delivery room. For those with the more traditional division between the two functions, a question frequently asked is, "When should the patient be moved to the delivery room?" The objective is to have the laboring patient in the delivery room 10 to 15 minutes in advance of the birth so that the delivery equipment can be prepared and so that the obstetrician can scrub. For women undergoing their first labors, the transfer should take place when the fetus is crowning, that is, when the scalp is visible through the labia between contractions.

Women with subsequent labors are much more unpredictable and should often be moved to the delivery room shortly after complete dilatation. Those with particularly fast labors might even be transferred when they are 8 cm dilated.

FETAL MONITORING

There are three important features of every tracing that must be assessed before the heart rate pattern can be properly interpreted. Each is defined below.

There are two techniques to monitor the fetal heart rate. External monitoring uses Doppler ultrasound to detect fetal heart wall motion. The internal method involves placing an electrode directly on the fetal presenting part to detect the QRS pulsing wave, as with a cardiogram (Fig. 6–1). This can only be done if the membranes are ruptured and is thus not appropriate for monitoring far in advance of labor.

Baseline

This is the central "beats per minute" (BPM) value that the fetal heart rate oscillates around for 10 minutes or more. The normal range is 120 to

Figure 6–1. Application of internal fetal electrode (IFE). (From Freeman, RK and Garite, TJ: Fetal Heart Rate Monitoring. Williams & Wilkins, Baltimore, 1981, p 47, with permission.)

160. A baseline of more than 160 is a tachycardia; if less than 120 it is called bradycardia.

Tachycardia may suggest fetal compromise but not invariably so. The <u>differential diagnosis of tachycardia</u> includes prematurity, maternal fever, minimal fetal hypoxia, uterine tachysystole, drugs (atropine), arrhythmias, and hyperthyroidism.

Variability

Long-Term Variability (LTV). This is an oscillation about the baseline that occurs with a frequency of 2 to 6 cycles per minute (Fig. 6–2). The normal amplitude is changes of 6 to 15 BPM (measured from peak to nadir of the oscillation).

Short-Term Variability (STV). This consists of beat-to-beat changes in the pulse rate from one

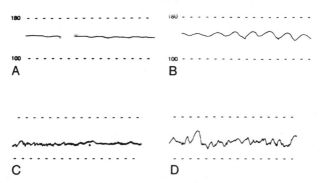

Figure 6–2. Short-term variability (STV) and long-term variability (LTV). **A,** Absent LTV, absent STV. **B,** Good LTV, absent STV. **C,** Good STV, absent LTV. **D,** Good LTV, good STV. (From Zanini, B, et al: Am J Obstet Gynecol: 136:44, 1980, with permission.)

moment to the next. The normal amplitude is 2 to 3 BPM changes. This cannot be measured by most external Doppler devices as they add artifact (every plot pointed is an average of the last three beats) that appears to be STV. STV makes the heart rate tracing look "jiggly."

Decreases in LTV occur frequently and are most often due to sedation. Fetuses also have so-called sleep periods when LTV is reduced that can be quite variable in length. Other possibilities include early hypoxia, drugs, prematurity, tachycardia, tachysystole, anomalies, and arrhythmias. Decreases in STV are less frequent than decreases in LTV. Complete absence of STV is cause for concern.

Periodic Changes (Decelerations)

(Umbilical cord compression)

Variable Decelerations. Variable in shape, duration, and timing with respect to contractions (Figs. 6–3 and 6–4). The heart rate can often drop

Figure 6–3. Tracing with mild variables. (Bottom portion represents contraction pattern.) (From Freeman, RK and Garite, TJ: Fetal Heart Rate Monitoring. Williams & Wilkins, Baltimore, 1981, p 71, with permission.)

below 100 BPM and even 80 BPM. One classification scheme is given in Table 6–1. It is thought that variable decelerations are a reflex response to umbilical cord compression.

Late Decelerations. These are decreases in the heart rate that are late onset, mirror contractions in symmetry, and are repetitive (Fig. 6–5). They may often be very mild in terms of amplitude change. <u>Cause</u>: <u>Uteroplacental insufficiency.</u>

As with baseline and variability, the interpretation of periodic changes requires experience and judgment. In general, the most ominous periodic changes are:

1. Repetitive, severe variables that are nonremediable.

Figure 6–4. Tracing with moderate variables. (Bottom portion represents contraction pattern.) (From Freeman, RK and Garite, TJ: Fetal Heart Rate Monitoring. Williams & Wilkins, Baltimore, 1981, p 71, with permission.)

Table 6–1. VARIABLE DECELERATIONS

DECELER-ATIONS	DURATION (SECONDS)		
	<30	**30–60**	**>60**
>80	Mild	Mild	Moderate
70–80	Mild	Moderate	Moderate-severe
<70	Moderate	Moderate-severe	Severe

2. Late decelerations that are nonremediable.
3. Prolonged, severe variables (lasting several minutes).

Intervention

1. Severe, prolonged variables
   a. Change maternal position
   b. Decrease uterine activity (turn oxytocin down)
   c. Oxygen
   d. Elevate presenting part

Figure 6–5. Late decelerations (also poor STV, poor LTV). (From Freeman, RK and Garite, TJ: Fetal Heart Rate Monitoring. Williams & Wilkins, Baltimore, 1981, p 68, with permission.)

e. Prepare for cesarean section (patient should have an intravenous [IV] line)
2. Late decelerations
   a. Decrease uterine activity (turn off oxytocin)
   b. Left lateral decubitus
   c. Oxygen
   d. Hydrate to expand blood volume
   e. Prepare for cesarean section
3. Cesarean section—The decision for immediate delivery on the basis of fetal monitoring is based on the periodic changes together with changes in baseline heart rate or variability. Nonremediable prolonged decelerations (for more than several minutes) or nonremediable, recurrent severe variables or late decelerations that persist for more than 30 minutes are often indications for prompt delivery.

Scalp pH

This ancillary tool can be helpful in interpreting equivocal tracings. The membranes must be ruptured and the cervix 3 cm dilated before a pH can be obtained. Two samples are obtained per effort, if possible.

pH >7.25: Reassuring.
7.20 < pH < 7.25: "Preacidotic" (consider repeating in 30 minutes).
pH <7.20: Delivery promptly.

Remember: Fetal monitoring more accurately predicts a healthy baby than a depressed baby.

The Limitations of Fetal Monitoring

New initiates to the world of fetal monitoring may be struck by the degree of disagreement among experienced nurses and doctors over specific monitor tracings. In fact, biomedical engineers have thus far failed to come up with reliable computer interpretations of monitor tracings, in contrast to successful programs written to interpret adult electrocardiograms. If you find monitor tracing interpretation confusing, do not worry: it is. The universal use of fetal monitoring in the United States is a prime example of well-intentioned research being misapplied. Fetal monitoring escaped from the lab due to bad science.

During the initial research with fetal monitoring in the early 1960s, certain types of pulse patterns were associated with fetal hypoxemia in both animals and humans. At the time, it was thought that many cases of mental retardation and even perhaps cerebral palsy were related to events that occurred in labor. Because the initial observations seemed to support this idea, the monitoring technology spread from high-risk research settings into general usage, but it is now apparent that the initial premise upon which monitoring was founded was wrong. Ninety percent of mental retardation and cerebral palsy is thought to occur before the onset of labor—the result of injuries sustained by the fetus over a period of time. Furthermore, among those few fetuses who are adversely affected during labor, a significant number experience sudden catastrophes that occur with little warning and leave little time for effective intervention.

In studies of fetal monitoring (started long after it was in widespread use), neonatal outcome has not been improved in low-risk populations. Furthermore, in comparison with populations in whom the nurse used brief periods of auscultation, the cesarean section rate increased. The initial premise was wrong, and in keeping with current knowledge, fetal monitoring in practice seems to be of no benefit in the general population. (A small group of women with significant medical problems such as hypertension, heart disease, or diabetes may be an exception.)

With these limitations in mind, why monitor? The most practical answer is that no one knows how do to anything else. As monitoring has replaced auscultation, there are no protocols about when to act with auscultation. Some obstetricians point out that it is also cost effective, as one nurse can remotely monitor several patients at the same time. I think the best reason to monitor laboring patients is that once in a great while, the tracing will suggest fetal intolerance to labor in a timely fashion. Particularly with a large number of women receiving significant interventions such as labor epidurals, continuous monitoring may yet be shown to have a legitimate role.

MECONIUM

This greenish substance consists of desquamated cells and other materials that accumulate in the fetal colon. The passage of meconium sometimes indicates fetal jeopardy, although fetal monitoring and scalp pH determinations have supplanted the importance of meconium as an indication of fetal well-being. More significantly, meconium in the airways can cause a potentially fatal pneumonia after birth. If it is thick enough, it may obstruct the airway and suffocate the newborn. As a result, the presence or absence of meconium must be noted whenever the membranes rupture (artificially or spontaneousiy). In most cases, the meconium is thin and does not prove to be a detriment to the neonate's health. Cesarean birth provides no protection against meconium aspiration. It is also becoming increasingly clear that there are other factors contributing to the neonate's illness in meconium aspiration other than the meconium itself.

In some medical centers, a pediatrician is asked to be available in the delivery room, particularly if the meconium is thick. The obstetrician should remove as much of the meconium from the oropharynx as possible shortly after the emergence of the head (even before the shoulders are delivered). This should be done both with the bulb syringe and some type of stronger suction device. However, the traditional notion that meconium "aspiration" takes place with the first breath of life may be oversimplified. With the increasing prevalence of the acquired immunodeficiency syndrome (AIDS), wall suction is beginning to replace the traditional DeLee trap for this purpose. It is possible (if not difficult) to inadvertently aspirate some of the baby's secretions through the DeLee trap.

PRESCRIBING PAIN RELIEF

Narcotic Pain Relief

The key principles in prescribing narcotics are not too early and not too late. If prescribed during a normal latent phase, there is some evidence that narcotics may prolong labor. (Paradoxically, a therapeutic "sleep" with narcotics may truncate a protracted latent phase.) Of course, if given too close to the time of birth, the newborn may have respiratory depression.

In practice, narcotics are not often given before the patient is 4 cm dilated unless sequential cervical change (indicating true labor) has been demonstrated. Keep in mind, though, that some

Table 6–2. EQUIVALENT NARCOTIC DOSES (FOR IM INJECTION)

Morphine	10	mg
Hydromorphone (Dilaudid)	1.5	mg
Meperidine (Demerol)	100	mg
Butorphanol (Stadol)	2	mg
Fentanyl (Sublimaze)	0.1	mg
Alphaprodine (Nesentil)	45	mg

women walk around for days or weeks at 4 cm. As a rule, if birth is anticipated in 1 to 2 hours, only an IV dose is given (if anything). If birth is expected within the next 60 minutes, most physicians do not administer narcotics.

An example of a commonly prescribed dose of narcotic is Dilaudid 1 mg IV push and 1 mg intramuscular (IM). Table 6–2 compares various narcotic potencies with morphine. The IV dose provides relief in minutes but rapidly wears off. The IM dose provides longer relief—usually for 1 to 2 hours. Sometimes a higher dose given more frequently than every 2 hours will be required. It seems that each subsequent dose of narcotic provides less relief than the preceding dose.

Demerol and Dilaudid both have peak action at 30 to 60 minutes after IM injection, although Dilaudid has a somewhat faster onset (15 to 30 minutes) and longer duration. Fentanyl is most useful as a fast-acting, short-lived IV agent. Alphaprodine (Nisentil) has been taken off the market by the manufacturer to reduce its product liability profile.

In the event that a narcotic is given close to the time of delivery, the newborn may have respiratory depression. If the baby is not breathing adequately, naloxone hydrochloride (Narcan) can be given IM, and the baby can be assisted for a few minutes with a bag and mask. The usual dose of Narcan is 0.01 mg/kg. As Neonatal Narcan is supplied in 0.02 mg/mL solutions for neonatal use, 1 to 2 mL IM usually suffices.

Narcotics commonly cause a decrease in the LTV on a monitor tracing. This fact is often used as a reason to withhold medication from women in whom there is some question about the heart rate tracing. It is important to keep in mind, however, that aside from causing respiratory depression following birth, narcotics are relatively safe.

It is worth noting that the maternal side effects of each of the drugs is largely the same, although some patients will be adversely affected by one and not the other. All narcotics can cause sedation and nausea. Bear in mind that patients will frequently confuse a side effect such as emesis with a drug allergy.

Epidural Pain Relief

Epidural anesthesia (the "Cadillac" of labor pain relief) is most useful for women in prolonged labors. Epidural anesthesia tends to provide much better pain relief and is helpful at the time of delivery as well. As with narcotics, it is thought that administering an epidural before active labor can prolong the latent phase. In practice, most obstetricians prefer to see their patients 4 to 5 cm dilated, although many will give the epidural sooner if the patient is already on oxytocin.

Although an epidural does not hinder interpretation of the monitor tracing, as can a narcotic, the epidural is not without fetal risks. In particular, maternal hypotension with a concomitant decrease in uterine blood flow can occur. It is thought that this can sometimes happen even in the presence of a normal brachial artery blood pressure. The decrease in placental perfusion can manifest itself as significant, repetitive fetal heart rate decelerations. Fortunately, maternal hypotension can be corrected by either increasing IV fluids or by administering ephedrine 5 to 10 mg IV push. (Normally anesthesia personnel prefer to order this.) Caution must be used in administering an epidural if there is significant doubt about the heart rate tracing.

There is considerable debate about the effects of an epidural on the time course of labor. Although many studies show no difference in time course when properly administered, some obstetricians remain skeptical. Redosing an epidural after the patient is completely dilated and ready to push (second stage of labor) is particularly controversial.

Epidurals can be redosed immediately prior to delivery. This provides particularly effective pain relief for the birth itself and is very helpful for forceps deliveries.

An alternative to intermittent epidural dosing is a continuous infusion. In general, the benefits of a continuous infusion include a steady state of adequate pain relief and the absence of the total numbness that frequently occurs after a bolus of the medication, which may interfere with pushing. Many anesthesiologists add a narcotic to the epidural infusion to provide better pain relief with less motor nerve inhibition.

PROGRESS NOTES

Indications

It is helpful to write a progress note whenever the patient is examined, given pain medicine, or otherwise has significant intervention or change in status. Whenever the physician walks into the patient's room, he or she should initial the heart rate tracing for documentation of the evaluation.

Content

A standard note on a woman in labor consists of:

1. Subjective: Her perception of contractions
2. Objective:
   a. Frequency of contractions (by palpation, tocodynamometer, or IUPC)
   b. Dilatation/ effacement/ presenting part/ station
   c. Statement about fetal heart rate and variability
3. Assessment: i.e., progress in labor, etc.
4. Plan: Pain medicine, continued observation, etc.

Chart Notations

In labor and delivery, there are several places to record exams. One is in the formal progress note section of the chart. Another is in the graph area where dilatation and station are plotted. Finally, the exam can be written directly on the tracing.

INDUCTION OF LABOR

Indications

There are a variety of reasons to induce labor. Three of the most common reasons are discussed here.

1. **Elective.** Occasionally, the patient will have a strong preference for delivery before a certain date, such as job relocation of herself or her spouse. Elective induction also becomes a consideration for women at term with a history of fast labors who have advanced cervical dilatation with the current pregnancy. In these cases, if the induction promises to be a relatively easy one, it makes sense rather than risk a delivery en route. In any case, there certainly are situations in which a "purely elective" induction makes sense and poses minimal risks.

2. **Premature rupture of the membranes.** Roughly 10% of women at term will break their amnionic membranes before the onset of labor. While 90% or so of these women will go into labor within the next 24 hours, the remainder will not. In some populations, particularly those women in lower socioeconomic groups, the risk of chorioamnionitis tends to rise over time. To prevent infection, many obstetricians will induce labor after some time interval if it does not begin spontaneously (e.g., 6 hours to several days, depending on the circumstances).

3. **Postterm.** In obstetrical parlance, this does not mean "past the due date," but rather at least 14 days past it. As the risk of perinatal morbidity and mortality begins to rise after 42 completed weeks, most obstetricians will deliver the fetus one way or the other between 7 and 21 days after the due date. Usually, this means induction of labor.

Cervical Ripeness

One of the chief drawbacks to induction of labor is that it does not always work. The key to predicting the success and time course of the induction is the state of the cervix, what obstetricians refer to as cervical ripeness. A semiquantitative method for assessing ripeness is the "Bishop Score" that was first described by Dr. Bishop in 1964. This score assigns 0, 1, 2, or 3 points to five categories (Table 6–3).

In his article (Bishop, EH: Pelvic scoring for elective induction. Obstet Gynecol 24:266, 1964), Dr. Bishop suggested that a score of 9 or more had a very favorable prognosis for induction of labor.

Table 6–3. BISHOP SCORE FOR ASSESSING CERVICAL RIPENESS

CATEGORY	POINTS
Dilatation	
<1	0
1–2 cm	1
3–4 cm	2
5 or more cm	3
Effacement	
<40	0
40–50	1
60–70	2
80 or more	3
Station	
less than −2	0
−2 to −1	1
Engaged	2
+1 or more	3
Consistency	
Firm	0
Medium	1
Soft	2
Position of Cervix	
Posterior	0
Midposition	1
Anterior	2

Currently, the chief relevance of this scoring system is to give the obstetrician some idea of the probability that labor will be easily induced.

For women who have a compelling need for delivery but an unripe cervix, there are two commonly used methods of "ripening" the cervix. The <u>first</u> is the insertion of laminaria, dried, sterilized kelp, that absorbs water and swells when placed within the cervix. The effect is to mechanically dilate the cervix 1 to 2 cm over 12 hours or so. A variety of synthetic substances for this purpose are now available as well.

The <u>second</u> method for initiating labor in a patient with an unripe cervix is the use of prostaglandin gel. UpJohn has recently released a commercial product in prepackaged form. The gel comes with an applicator that permits direct application into the cervical os. Up to three doses can be administered, 6 hours apart. It should not be given if the patient is already having frequent contractions, and oxytocin should not be used simultaneously. The gel often initiates labor as well as causing the cervix to ripen.

Method

The majority of women at term will go into labor within 24 hours of artificially rupturing the membranes (amniotomy). This is also known as surgical induction of labor. The alternative is to medically induce labor with oxytocin, an eight-amino-acid peptide produced by the hypothalamus and transported to and released from the posterior pituitary gland. The chief danger of oxytocin is overstimulating the uterus. Fetal compromise or even uterine rupture may occur. However, with fetal monitoring and computerized infusion pumps, these hazards are rare.

There are a variety of protocols using oxytocin to

induce labor. Virtually all of them suggest increasing the dose of oxytocin every 15 to 30 minutes until the uterine contractions are every 2 to 3 minutes apart. Some protocols start with an infusion of 0.5 milli-International Units (mIU) of oxytocin per minute, others start with 1 or even 2 mIU/min. There are also different ways of increasing the medication. Some hospitals double the dose at 15-minute intervals until 16 to 20 mIU/min has been achieved. Others increase it in either 1- or 2-mIU increments. In any event, it is unusual to require more than 20 mIU/min for a successful induction. Many protocols also call for either halving the dose of oxytocin or stopping it altogether in the event of significant fetal heart rate changes or tachysystole. Tachysystole may be defined as uterine contractions equal to or exceeding the resting period between contractions.

At the higher doses of infusion (perhaps 20 mIU and above) the antidiuretic properties of oxytocin become clinically relevant. If too much water is infused with the medication, water intoxication may occur with seizures and ultimately death. This is an unlikely complication, particularly with the limited amounts of oxytocin needed for most inductions.

Is induced labor more painful than "natural" labor? Patients almost universally think so, although the medical literature is somewhat more divided. It seems that because the endpoint for the infusion, contractions every 2 to 3 minutes, may be somewhat more frequent than the average spontaneous labor, induced labor may indeed be more difficult. However, such labors are also probably shorter and it may be that whether induced or spontaneous, the patient will experience the same total number of contractions. Although some data suggest that induced labor contractions have the same amplitude as spontaneous contractions, there may be a more rapid slope to maximum amplitude. It also seems fair to say that the latent phase of labor may be greatly shortened and that patients do not have a protracted prodromal period with which to gradually ease into labor. Also, in spontaneous labor, much uterine activity occurs outside of the hospital before the patient is confined.

PREMATURE RUPTURE OF MEMBRANES AND INFECTION

With premature rupture of membranes (PROM), the risk of chorioamnionitis increases as time passes. The risk is generally small and remains small even with the passage of several days. Also, chorioamnionitis is largely cured with the birth of the fetus and rarely leads to serious complications. However, Group B *Streptococcus* can cause serious injury to the fetus; the incidence of this disease is low, but it may be further reduced through the more aggressive use of antibiotics.

Group B strep infections can be classified as early-onset (within a week of birth) or late-onset. Early-onset disease is characterized by bacteremia, pneumonia, and meningitis. The death rate can be as high as 15%. Late-onset disease is typically manifest as meningitis.

The value of screening cultures is controversial because up to 40% of pregnant women will be colonized, and no professional organization is currently recommending treatment of all colonized women. Prophylaxis does seem warranted in specific clinical situations, including preterm labor, preterm PROM, PROM longer than 18 hours, a sibling affected by Group B strep, and maternal fever during labor. Ampicillin 2 IVPB every 6 hours is a widely used prophylactic regimen.

7

CHAPTER

Procedures Performed on Laboring Patients

ARTIFICIAL RUPTURE OF MEMBRANES

Indications

There are two primary indications for artificial rupture of membranes (AROM): induction of labor and placement of internal monitoring devices. Of women at term, 80% to 90% go into labor within 24 hours of ruptured membranes (spontaneous or artificial). AROM has not been shown to speed labor for women who are already contracting with reasonable frequency and strength (although it is often done for this reason). Science not withstanding, it is almost the universal experience of everyone who works with laboring women that rupturing membranes does indeed speed labor. In particular, women in second labors and beyond often seem to deliver very rapidly if their membranes rupture at advanced cervical dilatation.

Precautions

The incidence of cord prolapse (an obstetrical emergency requiring urgent cesarean section) is roughly 3 in 1000 among women laboring with vertex fetuses at term. This incidence can be increased by inappropriate artificial rupture. As a rule, the membranes should not be artificially ruptured if the fetal vertex is not already well applied to the cervix to help prevent cord prolapse. This is a different issue than fetal station, as the fetal vertex can be at a relatively high station but still be in good approximation with the cervix. Of course, sometimes AROM is the only way to obtain critical information about fetal well-being. In these circumstances, the largely theoretical concerns over cord prolapse are set aside.

Methods

There are two ways to rupture membranes:

1. Amni-hook. Identify and stabilize the cervix with one hand and snag the membranes with amni-hook in the other hand. Leave the examining hand in place for a few moments to detect any change in fetal presentation or station as the fluid leaks out.
2. The internal fetal electrode is very effective in rupturing membranes if the cervix is barely dilated or the membranes are tight over the fetal head. As the woman contracts, the membranes will be sawed through by the wire and the drainage of the amniotic fluid will be satisfactory. It may take several contractions to adequately assess the amount and color of the fluid, however.

INTRAUTERINE PRESSURE
CATHETER PLACEMENT

Intrauterine pressure catheter (IUPC) (Fig. 7–1) is useful when poor or abnormal progress of labor occurs. There are now two types of catheters. The traditional method uses a fluid-filled catheter inside the uterus, whereas the newer technique places a microelectronic pressure sensor directly in the uterus. This latter technique simply requires zeroing the sensor just prior to sliding it into the uterus (the illustrated directions are right on the package). The traditional fluid system is somewhat more involved and is described below. It takes 3 minutes to set up and about 30 seconds to insert.

Figure 7–1. IUPC placement. (From Freeman, RK and Garite, TJ: Fetal Heart Rate Monitoring. Williams & Wilkins, Baltimore, 1981, p 45, with permission.)

Directions for Insertion

1. With sterile gloves on, open a sterile drape between the patient's flexed and adducted legs.
2. Slide the catheter through the introducer in keeping with the curve of the introducer.
3. Draw up 20 mL of sterile water through the syringe provided and then flush the catheter with this syringe.
4. With one hand, identify and stabilize the cervix.
5. Slide the introducer (with the catheter in place) just beyond the edge of the cervix at 4:00 or 8:00. Try to avoid placing it directly lateral as the uterine blood vessels are near.
6. With the other hand, hold the introducer and feed the catheter through it until the black mark on the catheter is even with the introitus (at 25 cm). Slide the introducer back out of the vagina over the catheter.
7. Attach the stopcock to the end of the catheter, the pressure transducer, and the syringe. The flange points to the off position.
8. Attach a second stopcock to the other arm of the pressure transducer.
9. Flush the air out of the transducer with syringe filled with sterile water.
10. Be sure to plug the transducer into the machine. Fix the pressure transducer so that it is at the same height as the middle of the uterus.
11. Open the pressure transducer to the atmosphere and close the other stopcock to the catheter. Turn the "toco" knob until the pressure reads 0. Then press the test button. The pressure should jump to 50. This step and step 12 may differ depending on the brand and year of the machine.
12. Turn the system off to the atmosphere. Open

the other stopcock so that it is closed to the syringe—the pressure transducer will then be open to the catheter. Between contractions, the pressure should read under 20 mm Hg. Have the patient cough—the pressure should jump. Contractions will usually generate between 40 and 80 mm Hg of pressure.

13. Air in the catheter will tend to damp the pressure, as will particles and mucus. The catheter needs to be flushed periodically when it does not seem to be working.

SCALP pH

Directions

1. Be sure that there are at least two scalp pH cartridges at room temperature and that the machine is on for 30 minutes prior to starting. The machine should indicate "standby." Just before proceeding, slip a fresh cartridge into the machine, close the door, and wait until the machine reads "ready." This takes about 2 to 3 minutes after inserting the cartridge. This procedure may vary among machines of different manufacturers and years.

2. There are two possible positions for the mother to be in: supine or lateral decubitus with the buttocks flush with edge of the bed.

3. Open the kit and put on sterile gloves.

4. Slide the white, plastic, truncated cone into the vagina.

5. Have the nurse affix the light source to the cone.

6. Slide the cone in far enough to visualize the fetal scalp. Press to form a seal between the cone and the fetal scalp so that amniotic fluid and cervical mucus do not enter the field.

Figure 7–2. Fetal scalp exposed to hollow plastic cone; nick made in fetal scalp. (Adapted from Creasy, RK and Parer, JT: Prenatal care and diagnosis. In Rudolph, AM [ed]: Pediatrics, ed 16. Appleton-Century-Crofts, New York, 1977, with permission.)

7. With dry swabs, clean off the scalp.
8. Apply the silicone preparation with additional swabs. This helps the blood form droplets on the scalp rather than disperse.
9. Study the razor orientation on the long handle. Make an "X" in the fetal scalp with very firm pressure. This may have to be repeated as the scalp is often soft and edematous.
10. With a long capillary tube, dab at the blood as it wells up (Fig. 7–2). Holding the tube transversely, dip the distal end of the tube into the clay and hand the tube off to an assistant. The assistant should slide the capillary tube into the upright receptacle within the cartridge. The machine will provide a print-out of the pH within 15 seconds or so. A new cartridge

should be immediately inserted to prepare for the second sample.

11. Repeat step 10. Observe the site to be sure that the bleeding stops. If necessary, apply pressure with one of the swabs.

8

CHAPTER

Vaginal Birth

TIPS FOR THE UNINITIATED

There are many texts on the "surgical" management of a vaginal birth. Indeed, the public often looks at the unattended delivery as something of a medical emergency. I would like to emphasize that very little assistance is required for most vaginal deliveries (Fig. 8–1).

Novice Performing Delivery without Immediate, Experienced Supervision

The instructions in this situation are quite easy. Do not break the bed or table, but do encourage the mother to push. When the baby falls out on the bed between her legs, suck the mucus out of the mouth and nares, dry the baby, and double clamp and cut the umbilical cord. Tears can be repaired after the delivery of the placenta, which usually occurs within the next 20 minutes.

Active Intervention

As the baby crowns, gently provide counterpressure to prevent the head from popping out. If

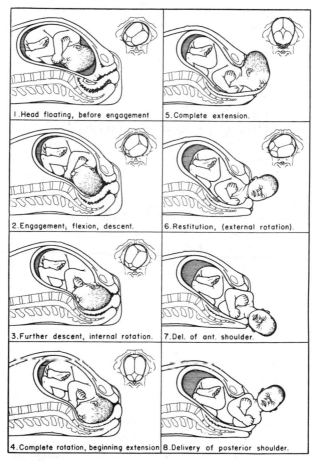

1. Head floating, before engagement
2. Engagement; flexion, descent.
3. Further descent, internal rotation.
4. Complete rotation, beginning extension
5. Complete extension.
6. Restitution, (external rotation).
7. Del. of ant. shoulder.
8. Delivery of posterior shoulder.

Figure 8–1. Orientation of the fetus through labor and birth. (From Pritchard, JA and MacDonald, PC: Williams Obstetrics, ed 16. Appleton-Century-Crofts, New York, 1980, p 397, with permission.)

a tear seems likely, inject 10 mL of 1% lidocaine in the midline, taking care to protect the fetal head with the opposite hand. Even with the injection of just local anesthetic, it is advisable to aspirate intermittently to be sure that the drug is not being given intravascularly. During the next contraction, use scissors to cut the episiotomy down the middle. If the scissors have one blade that is thicker with a rounder tip, use that blade within the vagina to minimize the risk of poking or cutting the baby. In some circumstances, the episiotomy should be cut off to the side (medio-lateral) to provide the maximum room.

Occasionally, episiotomies (and tears) can bleed quite briskly from small arterioles. Simply put a hemostat on these discrete bleeding sites before or after the baby is born. No benefit to mother or fetus has ever been proven from an episiotomy, although it is reasonable to make this incision if a tear seems certain. Repair of an episiotomy is often less uncomfortable than a more jagged laceration, which might need several injections of anesthetic.

As the perineum becomes increasingly dis-tended, keep up steady counterpressure so that the head eases out. Also, use a towel or a sponge with one hand to support the perineum in the midline. It is helpful to pinch the perineum together to prevent tears or extension of the episiotomy.

When the head emerges, allow it to spontane-ously rotate to face either thigh. Have the mother briefly stop her conscious pushing efforts at this point. Use the bulb syringe to briefly clear the mucus out of the nares and oropharynx. Before delivery of the shoulders, it is helpful to check whether the umbilical cord is around the fetal neck by sliding a single finger under the sym-physis and palpating the neck. If the cord is there, it can often be lifted over the baby's head. Alterna-tively, it can be double clamped and cut on the spot.

After the mucus has been evacuated, the patient should resume active pushing. Gently guide the

baby downward so that the anterior shoulder
delivers under the symphysis (Fig. 8–2). The fetus
should now be lifted upward so that the posterior
shoulder does not lacerate the perineum. With the

Figure 8–2. Delivery of anterior and then posterior
shoulder (with *gentle* traction). (From Pritchard, JA and
MacDonald, PC: Williams Obstetrics, ed 16. Appleton-
Century-Crofts, New York, 1980, p 421, with permission.)

delivery of the shoulders, the baby will slide out quickly. It is helpful to grasp the newborn firmly but gently by the neck and both legs. If the baby is reasonably vigorous, he or she can be placed on the mother's abdomen, before or after cutting the umbilical cord.

There is some controversy about where to hold the neonate in relation to the maternal abdomen and when to cut the umbilical cord. Some hold the baby below the perineum so that blood drains into the baby to prevent anemia. Others hold the baby above the perineum to reverse blood flow so that the newborn is not volume overloaded. It probably just does not matter for healthy babies. Also, the cord will stop pulsating on its own within a few minutes. Whether the cut is made immediately or with a delay is probably of little consequence. It is important to dry the baby off in the first few minutes of life and to keep him or her swaddled to minimize hypothermia.

Some institutions routinely request that cord pHs be obtained to help define the status of the fetus at birth. Double clamp off a 6- to 9-inch segment of cord, cut it, and hand it off. Arterial and venous samples can then be obtained with a heparinized syringe. For mothers with blood type of O or who are Rh-negative, an additional sample of umbilical cord blood should be obtained to determine the baby's blood type, Rh, and bilirubin.

SPONTANEOUS DELIVERY OF PLACENTA

This usually occurs within 20 minutes, although it can take longer. If the placenta is not out within 20 minutes of birth, an experienced resident should be made aware of the situation. Once the placenta is out, it should be inspected on both sides for completeness and the number of vessels in the umbilical cord. As long as the placenta seems to be complete, exploration of the uterus is unnecessary (in most institutions).

EXAMINATION OF BIRTH CANAL

Following delivery of the placenta, the cervix, vagina, and perineum should be inspected for lacerations. With a sponge stick in one hand, insert the other hand into the vagina applying downward pressure on the posterior wall. An assistant may also gently retract the anterior vaginal wall with an appropriate retractor. The cervix can either be grasped with ring forceps or blotted dry to aid inspection. If the cervix cannot be seen, it is acceptable to palpate it circumferentially to be sure that there are no major lacerations provided that there is not excessive bleeding. Palpation is often faster and less uncomfortable for the patient.

After evaluation of the cervix, the vagina needs to be visually inspected, particularly in the area of the ischial spines, as tears are not uncommon here. The perineum should also be inspected, particularly in the area around the urethra. A rectal exam should be performed to be sure that there are no tears in the rectal-vaginal septum and to aid with inspection of the episiotomy or other perineal tears.

A <u>first-degree tear</u> is a break in the skin or mucosa. A <u>second-degree tear</u> consists of a laceration that extends into the deeper tissues. A <u>third-degree tear</u> involves the anal sphincter, and a <u>fourth-degree tear</u> extends through the sphincter into the rectal mucosa. Superficial tears do not need to be repaired unless they have bleeding that does not abate with pressure and time.

REPAIR OF MIDLINE EPISIOTOMY

An episiotomy is not as easy to sew up as one might first think. As the fetal head emerges, it compresses the posterior vaginal wall into the perineum so that they form a single plane. Following birth, they resume their initial spatial orientation so that the vagina again forms a 60° angle with the perineum. The different planes and tissue layers can be confusing to those starting out.

The episiotomy can either be repaired with chromic (specially treated catgut) or Vicryl and Dexon (synthetic materials). All of these suture materials are absorbable. Chromic loses its tensile strength fastest—usually 50% by 1 week. On the other hand, it is usually gone by the time the woman resumes sexual intercourse. Some physicians suggest that there is more discomfort associated with sutures that dissolve faster.

There are four layers that need to be closed with an episiotomy. The steps below outline one approach among many.

1. **Vaginal mucosa.** A running suture of 3-0 gauge suture. This suture continues past the hymen out to the point where the tissue changes from pink to normal fleshtone. The suture is then not cut or tied but rather placed to the side so that it can be used subsequently (Fig. 8-3).
2. **Deep perineum.** The shiny white sheath of the bulbocavernosus muscles are usually visible on either side of the midline episiotomy. Three or four interrupted sutures of 2-0 material are

Figure 8–3. Reapproximation of vaginal mucosa (running suture). (From Pritchard, JA and MacDonald, PC: Williams Obstetrics, ed 16. Appleton-Century-Crofts, New York, 1980, p 432, with permission.)

placed in this layer. Substantial bites of tissue are included on either side of the incision, as this reapproximation provides significant strength (Fig. 8–4).

3. **Subcutaneous perineal tissue.** The 3–0 suture from the vaginal repair is brought out through the end of the repair underneath the skin. The running suture is then continued in the subcutaneous tissue in small vertical bites

Figure 8–4. Interrupted sutures in deep perineum (bulbocavernosus muscle). (From Pritchard, JA and MacDonald, PC: Williams Obstetrics, ed 16. Appleton-Century-Crofts, New York, 1980, p 432, with permission.)

(Fig. 8–5). It is tied at the end of the perineal incision if a subcuticular suture is not used.

4. **Subcuticular suture.** This is a running mattress suture beneath the skin edge with 3–0 or 4–0 suture. Some obstetricians use this, and

Figure 8–5. Reapproximation of superficial perineum. (This running suture can be a continuation of the suture from the vaginal mucosa repair. After this layer, the same suture strand can be used to finish the repair as a subcuticular suture.) (From Pritchard, JA and MacDonald, PC: Williams Obstetrics, ed 16. Appleton-Century-Crofts, New York, 1980, p 433, with permission.)

others do not. Those that do not argue that it is a waste of time, the perineum will heal just as well without it, and by placing absorbable suture just under the skin, the patient will experience more inflammation (and discomfort).

UTERINE ATONY

The most common cause of heavy bleeding after delivery of the placenta is uterine atony.

1. Massage the uterus firmly abdominally. If necessary, the massage can also be assisted with a vaginal hand.
2. Pitocin 20 to 40 mIU in 1000 mL can be run in at 200 mL/h (this may not be of immediate benefit).
3. Ergotrate 0.2 mg can be given IM. Preeclampsia and elevated blood pressure are relative contraindications to this drug.
4. Hemabate (carboprost tromethamine—a type of prostaglandin) can be given IM. It comes in vials of 250 µg. A common dose is 500 µg (two vials) IM. This dose can be repeated once.
5. Explore the uterus if heavy bleeding continues for more than 1 to 2 minutes and does not appear to be slowing. This should be done by an experienced obstetrician, as it is easy to miss a portion of retained placenta.
6. If these maneuvers are unsuccessful, reinspect the cervix and vagina for lacerations.

OBSTETRICAL SHOCK

There are no principles unique to obstetrics here, although patients can deteriorate very quickly. Signs and symptoms of shock include pallor, clammy skin, rapid and faint pulse, and in advanced stages, decreased mentation or even unconsciousness. Blood pressure, pulse, and urine output are all critical parameters. Blood should be drawn for complete blood count (CBC) with platelets and cross-match. Two large-bore IV lines should be established and a Foley catheter with a urometer placed. Junior residents should obtain immediate consultation. If a coagulopathy is a possibility, obtain a PT, PTT, fibrinogen, and fibrin degradation products.

THE DELIVERY NOTE

The protocol for documentation of the delivery varies. Some hospitals even require that a note be dictated. In any event, relevant information includes the following:

1. Type of birth (normal spontaneous [without forceps] vaginal birth—NSVD).
2. Obstetrician (who was present).
3. Type of anesthesia.
4. Estimated blood loss.
5. Delivery of the placenta (spontaneous or manually removed). Be sure to record it if the uterus is explored.
6. Episiotomy or lacerations.
7. Mother's blood type and rubella immunity.
8. The baby: sex, weight, and Apgar scores. If the cord gases are readily available, these too should be included.

The dictation that is mandatory in some hospital restates the above. If time permits, include a brief reference about the course of labor. Also indicate in the dictation a statement that the rectum was examined (and found to be intact).

POSTPARTUM ORDERS
FOR VAGINAL BIRTH

Most hospitals have a preprinted order sheet. Below are some general principles.

1. **Fluids.** Mothers who do not have an IV in place are often given 10 U of oxytocin IM to help the uterus contract and reduce postpartum bleeding. For those who have an IV already established, 20 U of oxytocin may be added to 1 L of crystalloid and run at a 6-hour rate for one or two bottles. The type of crystalloid used ranges from D5 0.2 NS to D5 LR. After a vaginal birth, the IV line can be removed when the patient is stable and eating, usually within a few hours of birth. The benefit of postpartum oxytocin in the absence of excessive bleeding or uterine atony is controversial.

2. **Vitals.** Every 4 hours for the first day. An example of guidelines for physician notification are for a temperature of 101°F or greater, a blood pressure of 160/100 or higher, and a pulse greater than 110. These suggestions are arbitrary and vary with each situation and patient.

3. **General diet.**

4. **Up ad lib.**

5. **Pain relief.** For vaginal births, Tylenol with codeine or Darvocet is often sufficient. An anesthetic spray (such as Americaine) may be ordered to help with episiotomy pain, as well as sitz baths. Some doctors order ice water sitz baths rather than warm ones for the first 24 hours.

6. **Labs.** A CBC on the first postpartum day is usually adequate.

7. **Rubella.** Mothers not immune to rubella are

traditionally vaccinated prior to leaving the hospital to be sure that they are immunized prior to subsequent conceptions.

8. **RhoGAM.** If the postpartum antibody screen is negative, RhoGAM is given to Rh-negative mothers with Rh-positive babies within the first 72 hours of delivery. Ten to 20% of patients who receive antepartum RhoGAM will have low antibody titers (i.e., ≤1:4) detectable postpartum. These mothers are still candidates for RhoGAM.

9

CHAPTER

Cesarean Section

HISTORY, INDICATIONS, AND TRENDS

In Caesar's day, a cesarean section was used to remove a dead fetus from a dead mother before burial. Prior to the late 19th century, it had at least a 50% maternal mortality rate. Over the past century, the development of improved surgical techniques, suture materials, blood transfusions, and antibiotics have made this operation a reasonable alternative to vaginal birth in some circumstances. The ability to deliver abdominally has probably been a major force behind the 100-fold reduction in the maternal mortality rate in the United States over the past century.

There are a variety of indications for cesarean birth. Common reasons include failure to progress, malpresentation (e.g., breech), fetal intolerance to labor, and maternal hemorrhage. Most of these indications are difficult to define precisely but generally fall into one of two categories: threat to fetal health or threat to maternal and fetal health. There are relatively few situations in obstetrics in which it is easy to say that a cesarean section is absolutely indicated. As an example, failure to progress may be appropriately treated with more observation, labor augmentation, or cesarean section, depending on the specific circumstances.

The cesarean birth rate in the United States has risen from roughly 5% in the early 1970s to approximately 25% by the early 1990s. There is much controversy in obstetrics about the appropriateness of this statistic. About one third of the increase comes from a higher rate of diagnosing dystocia or failure to progress. About 10% of the increase comes from the abdominal delivery of breech presentations, and perhaps 15% of the higher rate can be attributed to a growing propensity to diagnose fetal distress. Finally, approximately 25% of the increase in cesareans results from performing repeat cesareans, as there are more people who had the surgery in the first place.

One of the current controversies is the role of vaginal birth after cesarean (VBAC). The concern has always been about the integrity of the previous scar. If the scar breaks open catastrophically, a so-called rupture, the fetus can be lost and the mother can become quite ill. This is in contrast to the asymptomatic dehiscence in which the scar separates without causing symptoms. In the early 1980s, papers began appearing that indicated that vaginal birth after cesarean was "possible," that is, the mother survived the experience and an occasional baby was born vaginally. However, the real issue is the relative safety of VBAC versus elective, scheduled repeat cesarean section. By the late 1980s, papers were emerging that suggested that VBAC was actually safer than a repeat cesarean before the onset of labor. However, my own experiences and the subjective observations of many of my colleagues leaves room for substantial doubt. At this point, I regard the relative safety issue as unresolved. This is not to say that we do not encourage patients to attempt labor after cesarean. However, those who decline do receive scheduled repeat cesareans.

It is not clear whether the increase in the cesarean section rate is entirely without merit, although perhaps the magnitude of this rise might be questioned. The rate of difficult midforceps delivery has declined over the past two decades, and this may have played a role in increased cesareans over the same period. Perhaps some of the breech babies do benefit from surgical birth. In any event, the controversy over cesarean rates will no doubt continue for some time to come.

PREOP

Preparation

The following things need to be done to properly prepare a patient for cesarean section:

1. Nursing staff notified
2. Anesthesia notified
3. Written consent obtained
4. Magnesium citrate given (antacid)
5. Abdominal and pubic hair shaved
6. Foley inserted
7. CBC and type and screen sent off (sometimes anesthesia will want to wait until the results are back). This step can significantly delay operation if not performed well in advance.

Important Preop Considerations

1. Know the *blood type* and *hemoglobin*. Be certain that the blood bank did in fact receive the

type and screen (or sample for cross-match). The only time you will need the blood is when the blood bank did not receive it.

2. Know the location and reason for all abdominal *scars*—they will make a difference.

3. Know how much the patient *weighs* so that you know what to expect in terms of abdominal wall thickness. Pregnant women are difficult to judge in this respect.

4. Does the patient need prophylactic antibiotics? Certainly for indigent patients, *antibiotics* at the time of cord clamping should be considered for anyone who has been in labor with ruptured membranes. Before prescribing be sure you know her *allergies*.

5. Does the patient have a history of *fibroids*? When in doubt, just ask the patient. A strategically placed fibroid can cause enormous technical difficulties.

6. It may be helpful to check the last ultrasound report (if available) for *placental location.*

7. Know if the amniotic fluid has been clear or is *meconium* stained.

8. Be sure to check whether the patient wants a *tubal ligation*—this is easy to forget. Patients on public aid need to have special government papers signed 30 days in advance.

9. If the cesarean section is for cephalopelvic disproportion and the head is tightly molded in the pelvis, consider asking an *assistant to be available to help with the delivery by donning a sterile glove and pushing up from below if necessary. This requires preparation in advance. Often this can best be accomplished prior to the incision by gently pushing up on the presenting part to dislodge it slightly.*

10. Obtain the surgical consent. (See Chapter 10.)

OPERATIVE TIPS

Entering the Abdomen— Vertical Incision

1. Stay in midline and stay in site of previous knife stroke.
2. Make long, even strokes with knife.
3. Fascia can be cut with knife throughout. Alternatively, a small incision with a knife can be made and extended upward and downward with Mayo scissors.
4. The two rectus muscles can be separated bluntly for a primary section. Often scar tissue will necessitate sharp dissection on subsequent sections.

Entering the Abdomen—Transverse Incisions (Fig. 9–1)

1. Start at 3 fingerbreadths above the symphysis to minimize the chance of bladder injury.
2. Scarpa's fascia often looks just like the rectus sheath.
3. Once true fascia is identified, you may put the knife down for a moment and bluntly dissect off fat and Scarpa's. This is neater and quicker on primary sections but not always possible on repeats. Some surgeons do not like this blunt dissection.
4. Enter the fascia by making two small incisions on either side of the midline and gently connecting them with additional knife strokes using steady, even pressure.
5. Extend the fascial incision bilaterally with Mayo scissors
   a. There are two layers. They can be taken down separately or together by undermining first with scissors.

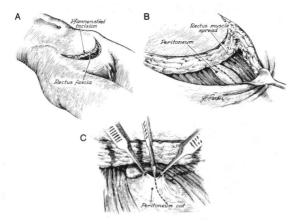

Figure 9–1. The Pfannenstiel incision. **A,** Skin incision three finger breadths above the symphysis. **B,** Rectus muscles exposed, separated in the midline and sharply dissected free from the overlying fascia, both above and below the incision. **C,** Incision into anterior peritoneum (entry into abdomen)—site chosen away from bladder at inferior aspect of surgical field. (From Wheeless, CR Jr: Atlas of Pelvic Surgery, ed 2. Lea & Febiger, Philadelphia, 1988, p 369, with permission.)

    b. The lower layer may be closely adherent to muscle (which bleeds if cut). Also, the lower layer attaches to muscle more medially than the upper layer—frequently the incision on this lower layer of fascia has to be curved upward to avoid this muscle at the lateral aspect of the incision.
6. *Mallard incision.* Cut the medial two thirds of rectus muscles transversely. Do not cut underlying, closely adherent peritoneum. Frequently the muscles are tightly adherent in the midline, and it is difficult to separate them bluntly—make a mini-Pfannenstiel incision (by dissecting the muscle off the fascia).
7. *Pfannenstiel incision.* After dissecting the mus-

cle off the fascia above and below the incision, the muscles can be separated bluntly or sharply in the vertical plane (harder to do on repeat section).

Entering the Peritoneal Cavity

1. Make the incision as high as possible on the peritoneal surface.
2. The incision for a vertical or Pfannenstiel is vertical; for a Mallard, it is transverse.
3. Dissect in layers when cutting through the preperitoneal fat.

Entering the Uterus (Fig. 9–2)

1. Make the incision in the vesicouterine peritoneum reasonably far away from bladder (not too low).
2. When dissecting the bladder off the uterus, remember that it is easy to poke a finger through the dome—keep fingers well applied to the uterine surface and go up and down— not side to side. If adhesions are dense behind the bladder they may be sharply dissected with Metzenbaum scissors, keeping the tips pointed toward the uterus.
3. The uterine incision should be 6 cm long and made in steady, gentle strokes. A lap sponge can be held in the operator's nondominant hand to keep pressure along the incision—this reduces blood loss over the incision and is more effective than aspiration in keeping the field dry. When only a few layers are left in the lower uterine segment, a single finger can be used to poke through. This "poke" should be straight through the wall—if it does not go through easily, more cutting needs to be done

Figure 9–2. Entering the uterus—sharp and then blunt dissection. (From Wheeless, CR Jr: Atlas of Pelvic Surgery, ed 2. Lea & Febiger, Philadelphia, 1988, p 219, with permission.)

with the knife. The incision should not be bluntly dissected as this often tends to dissect between the layers of the uterus and not through them, causing more bleeding.

4. The initial incision can be extended bluntly

with fingers or with bandage scissors. With bandage scissors, care must be taken to protect the baby with the nondominant hand (babies have lost fingers with this method carelessly applied). Also, the incision should be curved up as the lateral aspect of the uterus is approached to avoid cutting into the uterine artery. Many think that blunt dissection is faster, safer, and leads to less blood loss.

5. Occasionally, on entering the uterus, a sinus in the wall will be breached, resulting in heavy (and alarming) bleeding. In this case, do not panic or address that bleeding directly—proceed with the surgery. As the blood usually obscures the field, the assistant will do what he or she can to keep the field clean. As this usually is not perfect, you may have to proceed without ideal visualization. Remember to make the incision at least 6 cm long so that you do not dig yourself into a hole. If you cannot see midway down into the uterus, continue gentle strokes and palpate the remaining tissue between every two strokes. Sinus bleeding cannot be effectively addressed until the full thickness of the uterine wall has been incised and the fetus delivered. At that point, a single clamp is usually sufficient.

Delivery

1. Care should be taken that the hand is actually in the uterus. This may sound obvious, but the lower uterine segment is often thin and difficult to feel. More than one obstetrician has tried to deliver the baby with his hand outside of the uterus.

2. In delivering the baby, the hand should be under the head (sometimes a tight squeeze) before any upward traction is applied. The

wrist should be kept straight, and the lower uterine segment must not be used as a fulcrum because this will lacerate the uterus.

3. Fundal pressure is applied only after the head is within the incision.
4. If the maternal blood type is O or Rh-negative, the placenta should be delivered by massage of the uterus to reduce the fetal-maternal transfusion.

Closing

1. There are six layers that are usually closed: two uterine, parietal and visceral peritoneum, fascia, and skin. Some surgeons place sutures in a seventh layer, the subcutaneous (adipose) tissue.
2. For very heavy hemorrhage from a suspected laceration of the uterine artery:
   a. Use lap sponges to apply pressure to region of hemorrhage.
   b. Obtain second suction and advise anesthesia of greater than expected blood loss.
   c. Very slowly remove packs from lateral to medial to look for bleeding source.
   d. The uterine artery has to be ligated in two spots—low near top of cervix (in proximity to ureter) and high where it anastomoses with ovarian artery.

POSTPARTUM ORDERS

Vitals and Intake and Output

Vitals should be checked every 4 hours and intake and output every 8 hours for the first few days. An example of physician notification orders are the same as those for vaginal birth: a temperature 101°F, or greater, a blood pressure of 160/100 or higher, and a pulse greater than 110. Again, these suggestions are arbitrary and vary with each situation and patient. A physician should also be notified for output less than 250 mL in 8 hours.

Diet

This varies among physicians. Many will limit the patient to ice chips until the bowel sounds are active and then administer clear liquids. Patients are often not given a general diet until they are passing gas. In contrast, some obstetricians will place a patient on a general diet immediately, or clear liquids the first day and a general diet the second.

Activity

By the first postoperative day, patients should be ambulated (though they are often quite reluctant to get out of bed). *"Ambulate QID with assist"* is a good order for the first day. Immediately postoperative *"Turn, cough, deep-breathe every 1 to 2 hours while awake"* is also a good idea. For patients who received general anesthesia, the use of an *"Incentive spirometer every hour while awake"* to help prevent atelectasis may be a good idea.

Fluids

As a rule, 20 U of oxytocin are added to each of the first 2 L of crystalloid that are run at a 6-hour rate. The crystalloid chosen ranges from D5 0.2 NS to D5 LR. In practice, patients undergoing cesarean section are usually in good health, volume "overloaded" (from the pregnancy), and able to eat within 3 to 4 days postoperative. As a result, electrolyte balance, third-spacing, and precise volume replacement are not often of great concern.

Foley Catheter

A common practice is to remove the catheter on the first morning postoperative. Alternatively, the Foley can be removed a few hours after surgery. The logic for leaving it in overnight is to help the patient rest. Some obstetricians like to send off a urinalysis and/or culture and sensitivity prior to removing the Foley if the patient has not received prophylactic antibiotics.

Pain and Nausea Medication

Two methods of postoperative pain relief have largely supplanted the traditional IM injections of narcotics. The first, patient-controlled analgesia, entails the use of a computerized pump the patient controls. Whenever she is uncomfortable, she can press a button and receive a small dose of narcotics IV. The pump has a lock-out mechanism set by the medical staff that prevents the patient from receiving too much medication.

The second method is that of administering narcotics through the epidural catheter. This can be done on a one-time basis before the catheter is pulled postoperatively, or it can be continued by computerized pump for several days.

Patient-controlled analgesia and epidural narcotics require less total medication than IM injections, so they tend to provide a better level of pain relief with much less sedation and nausea.

For those patients who require IM narcotic injections, Dilaudid 2 mg IM can be ordered. Heavier patients will need more medication. These drugs and doses are examples of what can be used (also refer to the narcotic equivalency information provided in Table 6–1.) In the first 12 hours after cesarean section, the patient may not need much medicine if she has had epidural narcotics placed prior to the removal of the catheter.

Nausea can be controlled with Compazine 10 mg IM every 6 hours, Vistaril 75 mg IM every 3 hours (less often does not work well), or Phenergan 25 mg IM every 4 hours. Both Vistaril and Phenergan contribute to sedation and potentiate the effect of narcotics.

Antibiotics

Be sure to continue prophylactic or therapeutic antibiotics as indicated. (Some prophylactic regimens call for one or two postoperative doses.) Prophylactic antibiotics are frequently given for mitral valve prolapse as well as to reduce the chance of endometritis.

Miscellaneous Medications

When the patient is taking in clear liquids, the oral medicines below are commonly ordered. Every obstetrician has his or her favorites.

1. *Tylenol #3*, two tablets orally over 3 hours as needed for pain. Alternatively, Percocet or Percodan, one tablet orally every 4 to 6 hours as needed.
2. *Mylicon*, 80-mg tablets orally four times a day as needed for "gas pains." Mylicon will reduce

gastric indigestion but is of no benefit in abating pain due to small intestine peristalsis in the presence of colonic ileus.

3. *Halcion*, 0.25 mg (or Seconal 100 mg) one tablet orally at bedtime as needed for sleep. May repeat once. Although these drugs may appear in the breast milk in small quantities, the infant is rarely affected.

4. *Milk of Magnesia*, 30 mL every morning as needed or Colace 100-mg tablets orally twice daily for constipation.

Labs

Following a cesarean section, a CBC ordered on days 1 and 3 is usually sufficient.

Rubella

Mothers not immune to rubella are traditionally vaccinated prior to leaving the hospital to be sure that they are immunized prior to subsequent conceptions.

RhoGAM

RhoGAM is given to Rh-negative mothers with Rh-positive babies within the first 72 hours of delivery unless already sensitized (with >1:4 titers).

THE DELIVERY NOTE

The note should include the following (time permitting):

1. Type of cesarean section—both the type of abdominal and type of uterine incision
2. Preoperative and postoperative diagnosis
3. Surgeon and assistants
4. Type of anesthesia
5. Estimated blood loss
6. Mother's blood type and rubella immunity
7. The baby: sex, weight, and Apgar scores. If the cord gases are readily available, these too should be included
8. Any complications

EXAMPLE OF OPERATIVE DICTATION OF A CESAREAN SECTION

Name of patient—spell
Your own name—spell
Hospital number
Date of dictation and date of surgery
Attending surgeon
Assistants
Preoperative diagnosis
Postoperative diagnosis
Title of operation (be sure to indicate type of
        uterine incision)

Findings

At the time of surgery, the intra-abdominal contents, including uterus, tubes, and ovaries, were normal for a term gestation. A female infant with a weight of 7 pounds, 6 ounces, and Apgars of 7 and 9 was delivered from the left occiput transverse position.

Technique

The patient was prepped and draped in the usual fashion for a cesarean section. Under general anesthesia with endotracheal intubation, a vertical abdominal incision was made and the vesicouterine peritoneum was incised in a semicircular fashion over the lower uterine segment. The bladder was bluntly and sharply dissected off the uterus and retracted. A transverse incision in the midline of the lower uterine segment was made with a knife. The incision was extended upward and outward bilaterally with bandage scissors, taking care to protect the underlying structures with the opposite hand.

The infant as described above was then delivered. As the mouth and nares appeared, they were suctioned. When the rest of the baby was delivered, the cord was doubly clamped and cut and she was handed to the pediatricians who were in attendance.

The placenta was then massaged out of the uterus, which was explored and closed with two separate running sutures of 0-chromic, the second suture layer imbricating the first. With hemostasis achieved, the vesicouterine peritoneum was reapproximated using a running suture of 2–0 chromic. The gutters, ovaries, and tubes were inspected and the pelvis irrigated with warm normal saline. The parietal peritoneum was then reapproximated with a running suture of 2–0 chromic and the fascia closed using simple interrupted sutures of 0-PDS. The subcutaneous tissue was dry, and the skin was closed using staples.

The wound was cleaned and dressed. The patient was then awakened and moved to the recovery room alert and in good condition. The estimated blood loss was 800 mL. The sponge and needle count were correct at the end of the case. There were no intraoperative complications.

COMPLICATIONS

Although cesarean births may be common-place, the surgery has real risks. As a rough guide, the maternal mortality rate from vaginal birth is 1 in 10,000; from cesarean section prior to labor, 1 in 5000; and from cesarean during labor, 1 in 2000. Everything else equal, a laboring mother is four to five times more likely to die during abdominal rather than vaginal birth.

These statistics can be misleading, however, as they do not take into account the indication for surgery. For example, a woman who has cepha-lopelvic disproportion during a prolonged labor has a higher risk of morbidity and mortality without the surgery than with it. Because death is still an uncommon event, it is more meaningful to review the morbidity rate from cesarean birth.

Blood Loss

The average blood loss from a cesarean section is roughly twice that of vaginal birth—on the order of 800 to 1000 mL. Perhaps a recently marketed uterine stapling technique may cut down on the blood loss, but this has yet to be widely accepted as a fact.

Infection

This is by far the most common morbidity following abdominal delivery. In some studies, up to 50% of mothers will develop a postpartum endometritis. This statistic is very dependent on the length of labor prior to cesarean and the socioeconomic background of the patient. A wide variety of antibiotics administered in the perioperative period for one to three doses has been shown to reduce the endometritis rate in patients at high risk (long labors, etc.). Perhaps 1% of those with endometritis will go on to develop septic pelvic vein thrombophlebitis, a more tenacious problem requiring at least a week of heparin.

Damage to Adjacent Organs

Injuries to the adjacent bowel and bladder are not unheard of and can require additional surgery to repair. Rarely, even the fetus can be injured during the uterine incision.

Pulmonary Embolus

Although not a common occurrence, it is one of the most feared. As patients with abdominal incisions ambulate less than those with vaginal births, an embolus is more of a threat. This is one reason that early ambulation is encouraged.

Anesthesia

Even among the doctors, there is a widespread perception that regional anesthesia is inherently safer than general anesthesia. Not so. The mortality rate from both techniques is comparable and measurable in number of incidents per 100,000 (rare indeed). In the case of general anesthesia, the chief risk is from aspiration, whereas with the regional techniques, intravascular injection and subsequent convulsions and cardiac arrest are the chief problems.

10

Informed Consent

Many private physicians prefer to obtain their own consent. For residents who must obtain the consent, examples for cesarean section and tubal ligation are given below. In my residency program, it was a matter of policy to write in the chart that the patient knew that a tubal ligation could fail. As a resident, I wrote the discussion down in the chart verbatim, although most of my peers were content with the routine hospital form for surgical consent. This type of documentation cannot prevent lawsuits. It can, however, help to discourage them by showing the physician to be thoughtful and thorough. For those suits that are filed, a good consent can help your defense.

CONSENT FOR CESAREAN SECTION

The risks, alternatives, and benefits of cesarean section for_____ (give indication) have been explained to patient (and husband/baby's father). She (they) understands that the risks of cesarean section include but are not limited to:

1. Blood loss requiring transfusion.
2. Infection prolonging hospital stay and possibly leading to other complications.
3. Damage to organs requiring additional surgery (either at time of cesarean section or in second operation) to repair.

All of her (their) questions were answered, and she wishes to proceed.

CONSENT FOR TUBAL LIGATION

The risks, alternatives, and benefits of tubal ligation have been explained to the patient. She understands the following:

1. The surgery is permanent.
2. Once in a great while, the tubal ligation may fail and a pregnancy may result.
3. Pregnancy following tubal ligation has a high risk for being a life-threatening tubal pregnancy. She will see a doctor immediately should she suspect that she is pregnant following this procedure.
4. The risks of surgery include but are not limited to infection, damage to abdominal organs, and the need for a blood transfusion. (These complications are admittedly rare.)

All of her questions were answered, and she wishes to proceed.

11
CHAPTER

The Newborn

Although care of the neonate is no longer a major aspect of obstetrics, newborns will occasionally need assistance during the first few minutes of life. With this in mind, some basic information about caring for them is in order.

APGAR SCORE

Often misunderstood by parents, the Apgar score (Table 11–1) is a formalized system to assess the need of newborns for medical assistance in the first few minutes of life. It is most commonly obtained at 1 minute and 5 minutes of life. Apgar scores are notoriously unreliable for predicting the health of the baby after these first few minutes. Only a small minority of infants with 5-minute Apgars of 3 or less are neurologically abnormal at 1 year of age.

To judge muscle tone, merely move an arm or a leg and observe the degree of flexion. For irritability, scratch the soles of the newborn's feet and observe the response. The pulse is most easily obtained either by listening to the heart directly or by palpating the site of the umbilical cord entering the abdominal wall.

Table 11–1. THE APGAR SCORE

	0	1	2
Respiratory effort	None	Weak, irregular	Good, crying
Pulse	None	<100	>100
Muscle tone	Flaccid	Some flexion	Well-flexed
Color	Pale, blue	Body pink Extremities blue	Entirely pink
Reflex irritability	No response	Grimace	Cry

NEWBORN RESUSCITATION

What about intervention? The newborn should be dried off after birth and kept warm. As newborns have a relatively large surface area to mass ratio, they tend to lose heat very quickly. Keeping the infant warm during resuscitation efforts is particularly important.

Apgar 7 or Above

The newborn does not require any assistance.

Apgar 4 to 6

1. Continue stimulation by rubbing the feet, chest, or spine.
2. Be sure newborn is dry and warm.
3. Provide assistance with ventilation using 100% oxygen by face mask and gently provid-

ing breaths at the rate of 40 to 50/min. As the newborn has a small tidal volume, 6 to 7 mL/kg, the puffs do not need to be very large. To reduce the chance of pneumothorax, avoid using great force in assisting the baby with the bag and mask.

4. Continue observing the other components of the Apgar, particularly heart rate, color, movement, and breathing efforts. Most of the time, newborns will become more active within a few minutes of assistance.

Apgar 0 to 3

The neonate requires major assistance. When presented with a flaccid infant with few signs of life, most medical personnel experience a certain degree of anxiety. At this point, remember your ABCs—airway, breathing, and circulation. Even babies who are quite depressed at birth will usually perk up quickly with a few minutes of low-tech intervention.

1. **Airway.** It is a common tendency to suction the baby vigorously, particularly when it is not moving much. While not particularly harmful in itself, it interferes with providing breathing assistance. Except in the presence of considerable meconium, gentle suction of the nose and mouth for 10 to 15 seconds should be sufficient.

   More important than suctioning is the appropriate positioning of the neonate. The head should be gently hyperextended to relieve potential soft-tissue obstruction of the trachea (Fig. 11–1). This can be accomplished by placing a small towel roll under the baby's shoulders. It is not necessary (or desirable) to tilt the newborn's head as far back as it will go.

Figure 11-1. Position for keeping airway patent. (From Ostheimer, GW: Resuscitation of the newborn. In Ostheimer, GW [ed]: Manual of Obstetric Anesthesia. Churchill Livingstone, New York, 1984, p 337, with permission of the author.)

2. **Breathing.** As described above, 100% oxygen can be administered by bag and mask at the rate of 40 to 50 breaths/min. Again, the key word here is gentle—puffs of 20 to 30 mL should be sufficient.
3. **Circulation.** With a pulse significantly under 10 for any length of time, cardiac compression should be initiated (Fig. 11-2). Chest compression for the neonate is very different than that for the adult. It is faster and requires much less force.
   a. This should be done at a rate of 120 beats/ min.
   b. The sternum should be depressed 1 to 1.5 cm.
   c. Use the second and third fingertips over the middle third of the sternum, or both thumbs while gently grasping the thorax with two hands.

Drugs and Other Resuscitation Techniques

There are two other things that can be done to assist the newborn: intubation and establishment of IV access for medication. By and large, the

Figure 11–2. Neonatal CPR (two-thumb technique). (From Ostheimer, GW: Resuscitation of the newborn. In Ostheimer, GW [ed]: Manual of Obstetric Anesthesia. Churchill Livingstone, New York, 1984, p 336, with permission of the author.)

simple ABCs described above are sufficient for the first few minutes of life and, in most cases, all that is necessary. As intubation and IV access require some finesse and experience, they are beyond the scope of this book. Even so, a brief word is in order to give the junior house-officer an idea of the role of more advanced resuscitation.

1. **Intubation.** An endotracheal tube useful for the average term newborn is a Cole size 14 (with a tube diameter of 3.5 mm). A neonatal laryngoscope is required, and the head has to

be moderately hyperextended as described above.

2. **Circulatory access.** One of the most frequently used sites for obtaining access to the bloodstream is the umbilical artery. While not an entirely benign procedure, catheterization permits rapid administration of drugs and easy access for obtaining blood gases to monitor therapy. If the artery is too constricted at birth, the vein will occasionally be used on a temporary basis.

3. **Commonly used drugs and therapies:**

   a. *Sodium bicarbonate.* Useful for helping to reverse acidosis, the dose is 2 mEq/kg. It should be diluted with an equal volume of sterile water (with or without dextrose) and infused over 1 to 2 minutes.

   b. *Epinephrine.* Epinephrine is used to increase the heart rate and can be administered IV, IM, or by the endotracheal tube. For direct cardiac puncture, 1 to 2 mL of a 1:10,000 solution can be used. For the IV route, 0.1 mg/kg is suggested.

   c. *Volume expansion.* 5% to 10% dextrose in water or half normal saline at the rate of 100 mL per 24 hours. One bolus of 10 mL/kg may also be given. Alternatively, salt-poor albumin or even blood may be used (including blood collected promptly from the umbilical cord).

   d. *Naloxone (Narcan).* This is a particularly important drug for junior house-officers rotating through obstetrics. It can be administered IM and is contraindicated only in those with a known hypersensitivity to it (obviously not newborns). Mothers who receive narcotics too close to delivery will occasionally have depressed newborns. The dose is 0.01 mg/kg, so most newborns only require 0.03 to 0.04 mg. The reversal of narcosis is very rapid, with most newborns responding in 15 to 30 seconds of administration. It is important to keep in mind that naloxone has a relatively short half-life and can wear off before the narcotic has been metabolized. Since respiratory depression can occur again, babies given naloxone have to be watched more closely in the first few hours of life.

A BRIEF WORD ABOUT NEUROLOGICAL DEFICITS

Traditional thinking has held that cerebral palsy and mental retardation were intrapartum events and could thus be avoided. In recent times, the corollary was that if they occurred, the obstetrician must be at fault. Of course, nowadays, it is customary to sue one's doctor for these types of outcomes, and there are even expert witnesses available who will support such a contention, factual evidence or not.

It is now increasingly apparent that many cases of cerebral palsy and most cases of severe mental retardation are antepartum events having nothing to do with the course of labor and delivery. Unfortunately, as our understanding of these problems is still incomplete, most of these deficits are as yet unpreventable—electronic fetal monitoring not withstanding. Thus far, the biggest preventable cause of neurological damage is that of maternal alcohol consumption.

3
PART

The Postpartum Floor

12

CHAPTER

Daily Postpartum Rounds

FOLLOW-UP OF WOMEN WITH VAGINAL BIRTHS

Recovery Period

Women are currently given 1 to 2 days following birth to recover in the hospital. Their exam should include reference to breasts, uterine firmness and size, and amount of lochia.

1. After birth, the *top of the uterus* is commonly palpable at the level of the umbilicus.
2. *Lochia* (vaginal discharge) is generally bright red blood for the first few days and usually does not exceed one to two pads per hour. Clots greater than 50 mL are abnormal. The most common cause of excessive bleeding postpartum is uterine atony.
3. Generally the *episiotomy* does not need to be examined unless the patient has a fever or complains of severe pain in the region. The episiotomy may be seen by having the patient lie on her side, lift her superior leg, and viewing it posteriorly.

Discharge Checklist

Prior to the discharge, the following items should be checked:

1. **Temperature.** If the temperature is over 100.0°F in the last 24 hours, consider further observation. Examine the patient thoroughly for a source.

2. **Rh.** If the patient is Rh negative, be sure to know whether or not she received RhoGAM. One injection protects against 15 mL of fetal red blood cells. If her baby was Rh negative, she does not need it. If the mother had a large fetal-maternal transfusion (unusual and will be noted in the chart) she may need more than one injection of RhoGAM. This can be determined by ordering a Kleihauer-Betke (hemoglobin acid elution test), which can quantify the amount of fetal blood cells in the maternal bloodstream. Most obstetricians order this test only when a fetal-maternal transfusion is suspected, such as in the case of an abruption.

3. **CBC.** Patients are rarely transfused with a hemoglobin above 7 as long as they are not symptomatic.

Hemoglobin <9.0:	Ferrous sulfate 325 mg TID for 2 months
>9, <10:	Twice daily
>10, <12:	Once daily

   These are guidelines only and are somewhat arbitrary. Constipation may worsen with large doses of iron.

Instructions and Miscellaneous Considerations

1. **Sex.** Although many couples will not wait, it seems reasonable to advise abstinence for 4

weeks. While this is an arbitrary period, usually the vaginal lacerations and episiotomy will be healed enough to permit intercourse without great discomfort. Even so, most women will have at least some discomfort with the resumption of sexual activity. Also, some may notice inadequate vaginal lubrication. These patients should be reassured that this is a temporary condition that resolves within a few months. K-Y Jelly or other water-soluble lubricants may be suggested as an alternative.

2. **Contraception.** Some centers will start some patients on oral contraception on postpartum day 14. The delay of 2 weeks is to avoid the peak of hypercoagulability from pregnancy. An alternative is wait to prescribe the pill until the postpartum check-up. The pill should not be prescribed to breast-feeding mothers because it can reduce the volume of milk and because of concerns about exposing the neonate to exogenous hormones in the breast milk.

   For those who are breast-feeding or do not want the pill, the condom is the method of choice for the first postpartum month as the sponge and diaphragm have uncertain effectiveness in this brief time span.

3. **Driving.** While driving poses no inherent dangers to the new mother, she may pose dangers to others in the first few weeks. Those with significant episiotomy pain may experience a slight hesitation in using the brake because of their discomfort. Mothers who are anemic or very fatigued may not be as attentive as they should be while driving. It seems prudent to proscribe driving for the first few weeks, although the advice should be individualized.

4. **Bathing.** Tub baths can be very soothing for episiotomy repairs, and mothers should be encouraged to use them. For those with cesar-

ean section, many obstetricians prefer to avoid soaking the incision for 1 to 2 weeks after surgery, although there is no harm in getting it wet during a shower.

5. **Activity.** A good common sense rule is that "If it hurts, don't do it." The more patients move around in the first week or so, the more sore their episiotomy becomes, although activity will not slow its healing. For those who want to resume exercise, advice should be tailored to the patient's circumstances.

6. **Vaginal bleeding.** This can persist for 3 to 4 weeks, although it should not be heavier than a period. The passage of blood clots alone does not signify abnormally heavy bleeding. Women who have to change more than one or two pads an hour for several hours should call. It is reasonable to restrict tampon use for the first 2 to 4 weeks to allow the lacerations to heal and the cervix to constrict.

7. **Bowel care.** Most mothers are at least somewhat fearful of their first postpartum bowel movement because of constipation or the presence of stitches in close proximity to the anus. With the ever-shortening hospital stay, patients are frequently sent home prior to moving their bowels. Rarely, women can become impacted. To prevent this, mothers should be encouraged to take some sort of laxative such as Milk of Magnesia or Dulcolax (two tablets) on a daily basis until their first bowel movement. Those who do not move their bowels by postpartum day 5 should be encouraged to call the doctor.

Hemorrhoids are also a major source of concern, although they invariably improve at least somewhat with the birth. There are three steps for helping those with hemorrhoids. The first is to add fiber and fluid to the diet to reduce constipation. Simply increasing vegetables is usually not enough, and specific diet additives such as Metamucil or Fiberall may be more helpful. The second is to avoid traumatizing the area. This can be accomplished by minimizing wiping after defecation or through the use of soft medicated pads such as Tucks. Finally, rectal suppositories can be used after each bowel movement to ease pain and swelling. A good over-the-counter drug is Preparation H. An alternative prescription medication is Anusol-HC, on awakening and at bedtime (and after each bowel movement). This is a mixture of medications including a topical anesthetic and hydrocortisone.

8. **Pain medication.** Narcotic pain relief is rarely necessary after vaginal birth, although some women with particularly uncomfortable episiotomies will benefit from it. Acetaminophen with codeine (Tylenol #3), two tablets every 4 hours is often helpful. An alternative is 100 mg of propoxyphene with 650 mg of acetaminophen (Darvocet-N 100), one tablet every 4 hours as needed.

9. **Swelling.** Some women will notice increased swelling in their legs and hands during the first few days after birth. This is normal and is a result of fluid shifts following birth that resolve within a week by diuresis.

10. **Breast care.** See Chapter 13.

FOLLOW-UP OF CESAREAN SECTION PATIENTS

Progress Notes

The guidelines here are one approach to the documentation on a postoperative patient. For the first 2 days or so following cesarean birth, progress notes should include reference to the following:

1. Vital signs and urine output
2. Breasts
3. Lungs
4. Abdomen: bowel sounds/distension/tenderness/uterine firmness
5. Incision
6. Quantity of lochia
7. Lower extremities: tenderness, palpable cords, edema

Following the first 2 days or so, the notes can be less extensive as long as the patient is doing well. The abdominal exam and reference to the incision remain important.

Follow-up Labs

The labs usually obtained are a CBC on days 1 and 3 following surgery. Occasionally, a urinalysis and/or culture is obtained on removal of the Foley.

Special Problems Following Cesarean Section

Return of Bowel Function.   The large intestine is usually the last to recover following surgery. Bowel sounds are generated by the small intestine as the postoperative ileus resolves. The first signal that the large intestines are working is the passage of gas. Bowel sounds are usually reasonably active by 24 hours following surgery. Passage of flatus is variable but usually occurs between days 2 and 4.

Obstetricians vary widely in their approaches

toward feeding the postoperative patient. One common method allows the patient liquids with active bowel sounds and then a general diet following flatus. The IV is removed when the patient is tolerating liquids well, as long as she is not receiving antibiotics. Some obstetricians choose to feed their patients immediately with either clear liquids or a general diet.

Removal of the Foley. The Foley catheter is necessary only during the surgery to keep the bladder deflated. Also, many patients will have urinary retention during emergence from anesthesia. After this point, however, the longer the Foley is kept in, the greater the risk of infection. Generally, the Foley is retained for the first night after surgery to spare the patient the discomfort of getting up several times in the middle of the night to void. If the patient is not still on prophylactic antibiotics, it is often helpful to get a urinalysis at the time of Foley removal, and then send a culture (from a refrigerated sample from the catheter) if the urinalysis suggests a urinary tract infection.

Staple Removal. This process, universally dreaded by patients having it done for the first time, actually involves minimal discomfort and takes about 60 seconds. Obstetricians vary on when they want the staples removed, but a common approach is to take them out on day 3 for transverse incisions and on day 4 for vertical incisions. Most physicians place Steri-strips on the wound edges following staple removal. The patient should be advised that the Steri-Strips are not holding her together and that those that have not fallen off in 7 days can be removed by tugging at both ends.

Activity. Thrombosis is a threat to an immobilized postpartum patient. Women recovering from cesarean section should be urged to begin walking on the first day postoperative (up QID with assist). They may also practice coughing and deep breathing. Those at higher risk for atelectasis (general anesthesia, vertical scar) should be asked to use an incentive spirometer every hour while awake.

Fever. There are several causes of fever that must be considered following cesarean birth.

1. **Atelectasis.** More common in smokers with a vertical incision and general anesthesia, it can also occur in nonsmokers with a transverse incision done under epidural. Physical findings are usually not prominent, although they may include increased pulse and respiratory rate and decreased breath sounds over the posterior lung bases. Atelectasis is usually not a cause of a fever greater than 101°F for several days. Pneumonia must be considered should there be a high fever and prominent lung findings.

2. **Urinary tract infections.** These are not usually thought to be a cause of fever unless the kidneys are involved.

3. **Mastitis.** See Chapter 13.

4. **Deep vein thrombosis.** A serious postoperative complication, deep vein thrombosis can cause fever but is very uncommon.

5. **Endometritis.** This is one of the most common causes of postoperative fever, particularly after day 2 or 3 postoperative (See Chapter 14).

13

CHAPTER

Lactation

Obstetrics is prone to fads, and breast-feeding is certainly not immune. Two decades or so ago, bottle-feeding was the rage, and now the pendulum is swinging the other way. Breast-feeding probably does offer some modest benefits over bottle-feeding, but formula-fed babies certainly can and do thrive just fine. Perhaps the most important consideration in counseling mothers on feeding their newborns is to avoid instilling gratuitous guilt. Parenthood is filled with anxiety as it is, and pressuring mothers either to bottle-feed or breast-feed provides no benefit. For some working mothers or those quite anxious about it, breast-feeding will not enhance bonding.

BREAST-FEEDING

Breast-feeding has some health advantages when compared with formula use. First, it is probably superior to bottle-feeding in terms of transferring immunity and important proteins. Formula contamination and expense are also avoided. As formula is somewhat higher in calories than breast milk, breast-fed babies may be less prone to excessive weight gain. Finally, for the mother who enjoys it, breast-feeding does enhance her relationship with the newborn.

As for breast-feeding itself, the sooner it is initiated after birth the faster milk will come in. Frequent feedings, every several hours, are advantageous. In terms of technique, the baby should be held so that it does not have to strain for the nipple. Also, as neonates are obligate nose breathers, the breast tissue should not block the nares. To remove the baby from the breast, the mouth suction on the nipple can be gently broken by inserting a finger into the side of the baby's mouth.

It can take a few days for the baby to get used to breast-feeding, and mothers so inclined should be encouraged to persist. Babies normally lose up to 10% of their body weight postpartum, although they rapidly regain it. While many drugs can be excreted in breast milk, few of them pose a threat to the baby. Specifically it is acceptable to breast-feed with most antibiotics.

LACTATION SUPPRESSION

Patients who do not want to breast-feed may be prescribed Parlodel (bromocriptine) 2.5 mg PO BID for 14 days. It is effective in preventing breast engorgement that can be quite uncomfortable for several days postpartum. There may be rebound engorgement following discontinuation of Parlodel in a minority of women. Alternatively, breast engorgement will resolve within a week or so postpartum and can be hastened with a tight bra and ice packs held to the breast. Parlodel may cause hypotension and should be given with care to patients who are significantly anemic. A recent advisory mailed out by the company that makes Parlodel warned of a possible association of stroke and use of the drug for lactation suppression. The company suggested that if there were a risk, it was a small one and stated that the subject was under study.

BREAST ENGORGEMENT AND MASTITIS

There is debate about whether severe breast engorgement can cause a low-grade temperature. It is rarely a cause of spiking fevers above 101°F. In contrast, if there is localized warmth, tenderness, and erythema in one breast, mastitis is a possibility, although this often occurs several weeks postpartum, after the patient has been discharged.

Patients with mastitis should be advised to continue breastfeeding and use warm packs and acetaminophen to ease their discomfort. While the milk itself can be cultured and Gram-stained, this is not always necessary in patients with characteristic findings. The bacteria often enter the breast through a cracked nipple. Common pathogens include *S. aureus*, betahemolytic streptococci, *E. coli*, and *H. influenzae*.

The initial antibiotic of choice is either penicillin 250 mg or dicloxacillin 125 mg four times a day for 1 week. The penicillin is cheaper, but dicloxacillin is effective for penicillin-resistant staphylococci. For those allergic to penicillin, 250 mg of erythromycin four times a day may be used.

Those who are not significantly better within 48 hours should be examined for a breast abscess. These frequently require incision and drainage. Early administration of antibiotics is usually effective in preventing this complication.

14

Postpartum Endometritis

RISK FACTORS

In some populations, as many as 50% of women undergoing cesarean section during labor have postoperative endometritis, although this number can be reduced to 20% or even lower with the appropriate use of prophylactic antibiotics. Endometritis following vaginal birth is much less frequent—on the order of 1%, and these infections tend to be less severe.

DIAGNOSIS

This most common cause of sustained postoperative fever is a diagnosis of exclusion. There are no reliable physical or laboratory findings that are completely diagnostic of endometritis. The uterus is always tender following cesarean section, and lochia can be foul-smelling even without significant infection. The white count can be elevated up to 20,000 following cesarean section done during labor in the absence of endometritis.

The common practice is to exclude other causes of fever and then to initiate antibiotics. Often, with a temperature spike, obstetricians will draw blood cultures from two separate sites and obtain a urine culture prior to starting antibiotics, though these rarely show bacteria. Lochia cultures are not usually of benefit. A CBC obtained within 24 hours of the first fever spike (before or after) is often sufficient. A differential adds expense and is rarely of diagnostic benefit.

When microbes are recovered, common isolates include the aerobes *E. coli*, Group B betahemolytic streptococci, enterococci, and the anaerobes such as *Peptostreptococcus*, *Chlamydia*, and a variety of *Bacteroides* species.

TREATMENT

The most thoroughly tested and effective regimen for postpartum endometritis is a combination of clindamycin (900 mg every 8 hours) and gentamicin (1.5 mg/kg every 8 hours). This treatment covers a wide variety of likely pathogens, such as Gram-negative bacilli and anaerobes such as *Bacteroides*. In patients who do not respond or for those who are severely ill, a penicillin might be considered for coverage against Group D streptococci (enterococci).

As a two-drug therapy, gentamicin and clindamycin seem to be superior to ampicillin and gentamicin. Other regimens have not been tested as thoroughly. Alternative treatment includes single-agent therapy with a second-generation cephalosporin or with a third-generation penicillin (mezlocillin 3 g every IVPB every 4 hours). Third-generation penicillins kill both Group D streptococci and *Bacteroides fragilis*.

With gentamicin, some physicians obtain peak and trough levels around the third or fourth dose. If there is a question about impaired renal function, checking a BUN and creatinine before or shortly after starting treatment might be a good idea.

A recently introduced antibiotic, Primaxin, seems to be a good first choice as an alternative to multiple drug therapy. A 1:1 mixture of imipenem and cilastatin, it kills a broad range of pathogens, including *Bacteroides* and *Staphylococcus* species. The usual dose is 500 mg IV piggyback every 6 hours.

Pseudomembranous colitis can be a problem with any antibiotic. Diarrhea consisting of several loose stools per day warrants sending off a stool sample for *C. difficile* toxin and culture, although the drug can be continued pending the results if the patient is not toxic.

There is one clinical sign that carries weight over all others in determining the response to therapy—the maximum temperature (T-max) in a 24-hour period. As long as this value begins to drop within 48 hours of initiating therapy, the antibiotic regimen is not changed. If T-max is not improving after 48 hours of maximal antibiotic therapy, abscess or septic pelvic vein thrombosis becomes a concern. These are both quite rare.

As a rule, the drugs are continued for a total of 4 to 5 days and for 24 to 48 hours after defervescence (depending on response and severity of infection). Although it is common practice in some institutions to discharge patients with a course of additional, oral antibiotics, the benefit of this treatment is controversial and should be individualized.

SEPTIC PELVIC VEIN THROMBOSIS AND PELVIC ABSCESS

If a postoperative fever fails to respond to appropriate antibiotics, and a pelvic exam does not suggest an abscess, heparin is usually started. 5000 or 10,000 U are given in 1 hour as a bolus and then 1000 U/h with subsequent dose titration based on obtaining a PTT every 4 hours until it is one and a half to two times longer than the control. If the patient responds, the heparin is continued for 7 to 10 days and then stopped without additional anticoagulation. There is significant controversy about discontinuing anticoagulation completely in these circumstances. Also, septic deep venous thrombosis should be distinguished from clots arising without prior infection in this circumstance, as most obstetricians would continue anticoagulation for several months with warfarin.

If the T-max does not begin to drop within 48 hours of heparin, then an abscess must be reconsidered. Obstetricians prefer to obtain ultrasounds to assist with this diagnosis, although in my experience, this test is of little value in either identifying or excluding an abscess. I think that the CT scan (which costs three times as much) is much more helpful. A pelvic abscess that does not respond to antibiotic treatment requires surgical drainage (extremely rare).

15
CHAPTER

Circumcision

INDICATIONS AND CONTRAINDICATIONS

There is no true medical indication for a circumcision as there is no clearly established health benefit from the procedure. Parents will request a circumcision for a variety of social and religious reasons. Most commonly if the father has been circumcised, the parents will request that their boy also have his foreskin removed.

There are some contraindications to the procedure. Hypospadias, significant jaundice, or a bleeding disorder in the parents requires the obstetrician to reconsider the surgery and consult the pediatricians before proceeding.

INFORMED CONSENT

The degree of formal consent obtained before this brief, "simple" procedure varies among doctors. It is important to emphasize the optional nature of circumcision, particularly as some patients believe that the surgery is medically recommended.

ANESTHESIA

An article in the *Journal of the American Medical Association* recently pointed out the safety and efficacy of administering local anesthesia in advance of circumcision. Whatever the evidence presented in *JAMA*, many doctors will no doubt view it as a waste of time with little benefit. Admittedly, it seems difficult sometimes to notice the difference, because many babies still cry quite vigorously, anesthetic or not.

Controversy or not, the technique calls for injections of 0.2 to 0.4 mL of 1% lidocaine at the base of the penis at 2:00 and at 10:00 near the course of the two dorsal nerves of the penis. Prior to the injections, the skin at the base of the penis should be stabilized with gentle traction. Ideally, the needle should be advanced 2 to 5 mm through the skin in a posteromedial direction. Before administering the lidocaine, the syringe should be aspirated to be sure the needle is not intravascular. The lidocaine should be without epinephrine, and no more than 0.8 mL should be given.

The practical result of these injections is that two small, practically contiguous blebs will form at the base of the penis. Anesthesia should be achieved within 2 to 3 minutes.

PROCEDURE

The circumcision takes only 5 to 10 minutes, but like the episiotomy, it is not as easy as it first looks. I will describe a procedure that uses the bell clamp. It comes in three sizes: 1.1, 1.3, and 1.5 (small, medium, and large).

1. Strap the baby into the specially designed tray. It is important to be sure the Velcro straps are attached above the knee to minimize the infant's kicking.
2. Put on your hat and mask, scrub, and put on gloves. The procedure is not as strictly sterile as an intra-abdominal operation.
3. Wash the penis off with antiseptic and drape the area. Administer the lidocaine at this point if you plan to do so.
4. Grasp the foreskin at 11:00 and 1:00 with two hemostats. The urethral meatus is difficult to find, as the foreskin is somewhat folded over it. By grasping the foreskin in approximately the right location with hemostats and then applying gentle upward traction, you can confirm that you have appropriate placement of the hemostats.
5. Slide a closed hemostat oriented transversely just underneath the foreskin at 12:00. Be careful to keep the tips pointed outward, away from the penis itself. Advance gently until resistance is encountered. Spread the tips and withdraw slowly. This serves to free up any loose adhesions between the foreskin and the glans penis. As the hemostat is being withdrawn, the glans can be visualized to confirm the anatomy. This step can be repeated several times until the foreskin slides more easily along the glans.
6. Clamp the foreskin with the hemostat at 12:00. The tips of the hemostat should be even with the bottom of the glans. Allow the clamp to remain on the skin for 30 seconds or so.
7. Cut along the foreskin at 12:00 with a scissors

in the groove created by the clamp. The bleeding should be minimal as the clamping step crushes the larger blood vessels.

8. With the help of the hemostats still affixed at 11:00 and 1:00, slide the foreskin back below the glans. This step further breaks up adhesions. I try to avoid the use of any instruments to vigorously break these attachments as they can bleed, but gentle, blunt dissection is often necessary. In particular, the skin at 6:00 attaches relatively high on the glans. Do not mistake this for an adhesion as this can bleed vigorously when disrupted.

9. Insert the appropriately sized bell under the foreskin and over the glans. It is helpful to use a third hemostat at 12:00 to pinch the foreskin together at the base of the bell to prevent it from sliding out.

10. Remove the hemostats at 11:00 and 1:00.

11. Take the flat base of the clamp and slide the bell portion through the hole at the end of the base. Gently affix the two prongs at the top of the bell protector to the receptacle on the clamp.

12. Look below the base of the clamp at the penis. The outline of the glans should be faintly discernible. Be sure that the skin here is not too taut or loose. Small adjustments in the amount of foreskin can be made at this point by gently pushing the tissue up or down through the loose clamp arrangement with a 2 × 2 gauze.

13. Tighten the large nut at the end of the clamp. This pulls the bell up against the clamp. This step is irreversible, as it crushes the blood vessels. It is important to be sure that the nut is turned as tightly as possible, as hemostasis depends on this step.

14. Some obstetricians like to wait for 5 minutes with the clamp on to be sure that hemostasis

has been achieved, but 1 to 2 minutes may be all that is necessary. I use a knife blade without a handle to cut off the foreskin *distal* to the clamp (above). It is important to get all the foreskin off and leave smooth edges. Otherwise the circumcision will leave a ragged edge of skin around the glans.

15. Loosen the clamp and gently slide the bell off the penis. Bleeding should be minimal. Should bleeding persist from specific arterioles, silver nitrate on a wooden applicator can be gently applied to the site for hemostasis.

16. Dress the wound with Vaseline and then dry gauze. Some hospitals have a policy that the baby is not discharged from the hospital until he urinates.

A FEW LAST WORDS

During residency, I learned several important principles with regard to this surgery. First, you only have one chance to do it right. Do not attempt to take off just a "little bit more" as this can be more difficult than it would appear. Second, it is sometimes difficult to tell how much is enough and not too much. As a rule, you want the skin of the penis to end at the glans. It rarely will. More commonly it will end a millimeter or so above or below the glans. Either case is an acceptable result. Finally, the penis can look amazingly bad the day after a properly performed procedure. It is typically black and blue and edematous.

4

PART

*Less Common
Problems*

16
CHAPTER

Preeclampsia

The junior resident's exposure to patients with preeclampsia spans the antepartum clinic, labor and delivery, and the postpartum floor. Because the clinical circumstances in which the disease is encountered are so variable, this chapter is organized by epidemiology, diagnosis, and treatment, rather than by geographic location of the patient within the hospital.

RISK FACTORS

1. First pregnancy
2. Extremes of age
3. Multiple pregnancy
4. Poverty (?)

DEFINITIONS

The diagnosis of preeclampsia is based on the finding of hypertension accompanied either by proteinuria or edema, or both.

Hypertension

Hypertension is diagnosed if one or more of the following criteria are present:

1. Diastolic ≥ 90
2. Systolic ≥ 140
3. Mean arterial pressure ≥ 105 (systolic BP + 2 × diastolic BP)/3
4. Rise in systolic of 30
5. Rise in diastolic of 15

Proteinuria

More than 300 mg in 24 hours. As a practical rule, 2+ protein on a catheterized urinalysis is diagnostic of proteinuria in the absence of a urinary tract infection. A 2+ protein in the urine on a dipstick always raises a question about preeclampsia in a pregnant woman. This can also result from leaking amniotic fluid or an infection in the vagina or bladder. Such a finding must always be checked with a catheterized urinalysis if the cause is not clear.

Edema

Clinically evident swelling (not too helpful, as 75% of pregnant women could qualify).

SEVERE PREECLAMPSIA

This can be quite a serious illness and is diagnosed when one of the following is present:

1. Systolic ≥ 160
2. Diastolic ≥ 110

3. Oliguria (500 mL or less in 24 hours)
4. Proteinuria of 5 g or more in 24 hours (alternatively, 3+ or 4+ on qualitative dipstick several hours apart)
5. Cerebral or visual disturbances (severe)

Many people make much of testing for reflexes in preeclamptics. It is important to keep in mind that the presence or absence of hyperreflexia is often hard to judge and does not contribute to the diagnosis of preeclampsia (unless extreme). However, sustained clonus can be a worrisome finding in a patient who already has the diagnosis of preeclampsia. Central nervous system irritability is associated with increased risk for seizure but is not 100% predictive.

6. Epigastric pain (can signal hepatic edema)
7. Pulmonary edema or cyanosis
8. Thrombocytopenia
9. Intrauterine growth retardation (see Chapter 17)

ECLAMPSIA

This is the occurrence of a seizure in a preeclamptic patient not attributable to other causes. Seizures can occur up to 1 week following delivery, but the period of highest risk ends after the first 24 hours following birth.

LABORATORY EVIDENCE

Usually, there are few laboratory abnormalities in preeclamptic patients because most patients develop the illness close to term and do not become very ill. An SMA-20, CBC with platelets, and occasionally a PT, PTT, fibrinogen, and fibrin degradation products should be drawn. For patients in labor, it is also prudent to send a type and screen in the event that cesarean section becomes necessary. Things to look for include:

1. Increased (or even normal) hemoglobin. This can suggest hemoconcentration as vascular permeability increases and fluid begins to "third space."
2. Uric acid > 5.5.
3. Creatinine > 1 (not completely reliable).
4. BUN > 10 (not completely reliable).
5. Colloid oncotic pressure. Not a very useful clinical marker, this value drops in some preeclamptics.
6. Thrombocytopenia. In up to 20% of severe preeclamptics, the platelet count can be decreased. Although disseminated intravascular coagulation (DIC) can occur in preeclampsia, it is rather uncommon—particularly in the face of a normal platelet count.

TREATMENT

Preeclampsia is cured with the delivery of the fetus and always worsens the longer the pregnancy continues. At term, the first principle of treatment is delivery. Preterm, the decision is more difficult as the fetus may also be in jeopardy from premature birth. Severe preeclamptics are commonly delivered promptly at any gestational age.

Seizure Prophylaxis

Begin with 4 to 6 g magnesium sulfate IV piggyback over 20 minutes and continue it at 2 g/h. If deep tendon reflexes are brisk or clonus persists, the dose can be raised, usually in 0.5 to 1 g/h increments. Magnesium takes 12 to 18 hours to equilibrate, rendering magnesium levels of dubious benefit, because infusions rarely go longer than 2 days. The therapeutic level is considered to be between 4 and 8 mEq/L. Magnesium is cleared by the kidneys, and its level will climb with poor urine output. At levels of 10 to 12 mEq and above, muscle weakness, respiratory paralysis, and cardic depression can ensue. Calcium gluconate should be administered IV in the event of magnesium toxicity. Seizures can occur even with "therapeutic" levels of magnesium.

To significantly decrease the level of magnesium in the bloodstream it is more effective to stop the drug for 1 to 2 hours rather than simply to turn the infusion down. Similarly, repeated boluses (2 g over 10 minutes) can be given to raise the level along with increasing the steady infusion rate.

The magnesium infusion is usually stopped 24 hours postpartum. While the magnesium infusion is continued, respirations and urine output are checked every hour (this requires a Foley). Deep tendon reflexes can serve as a rough guide to magnesium levels. When they are significantly decreased, the dose should probably not be raised.

Ordering a "toxemia protocol" in most hospitals is sufficient to indicate the need for hourly observation. Magnesium has killed hospitalized patients in the past through overdosage leading to respiratory depression. This can occur if the magnesium infusion runs in wide open without an infusion pump.

In rabbits, magnesium can lower the diastolic blood pressure by as much as 10 mm Hg. In humans, this effect is less clear. If magnesium does have a beneficial impact on blood pressure, it is a small one.

Magnesium can cause a modest decrease in fetal heart rate variability. It is important to remember that fetuses in preeclamptic mothers are in some jeopardy in the first place and their tracings have to be reviewed carefully.

Blood Pressure Control

When the diastolic blood pressure climbs to 110 or above, the possibility of intracerebral hemorrhage increases, and medication is indicated. Hydralazine (Apresoline) 5 to 10 mg IV push is the drug of choice. The onset of effect is 10 to 20 minutes with a maximum effect at 20 to 40 minutes. If no response is seen in 15 minutes or so, the dose can be repeated. If three doses per hour are needed to keep the diastolic under 110, an Apresoline drip beginning at 1 mg/h can be initiated. It is critical not to lower the blood pressure too precipitously, as this can be harmful to both mother and fetus. Diastolic blood pressures under 105 usually are not treated.

Oliguria

This is often the most vexing problem in severe preeclamptics, as there is no clearly preferable course of treatment. The patient is already predisposed to pulmonary edema and is very sensitive to fluid challenges. Paradoxically, the patient is also intravascularly volume depleted.

As a rule, patients with oliguria intrapartum warrant a central line to aid fluid replacement. A Swan-Ganz catheter is preferable, as there can be significant right-left cardiac dysfunction. Preeclamptics have an excess of total body sodium but are intravascularly depleted. Thus, some obstetricians argue for replacement with

0.2 normal saline (NS), whereas others insist on 0.9 NS. In the United States, the use of Lasix to maintain urine output is discouraged, although in Britain it is quite commonly used. Again, central line monitoring can be quite helpful in guiding therapy.

17

CHAPTER

Twins

INCIDENCE AND CAUSE

In a discussion of twins, a distinction should be made from the outset between monozygotic and dizygotic siblings. The frequency of monozygotic (identical) twinning is constant throughout the world and occurs at the rate of approximately 4 per 1000 pregnancies. In contrast, dizygotic (fraternal) twins occur at variable rates:

Asians	2/1000 pregnancies
White Americans	6/1000
Black Americans	10/1000
Blacks (Nigeria)	40/1000

As can be seen, this highly variable dizygotic twinning rate influences the percentage of monozygotic twins born within a given population. For instance, two thirds of Asian twins are identical, while only 1 of every 10 twins born in Nigeria are monozygotic.

The differing epidemiology between the two types of twins suggests a different cause as well. While the cause of embryo cleavage within 14 days of conception is poorly understood, identical twinning tends to be a randomly occurring event independent of family history and other factors. In sharp contrast, dizygotic twinning is related directly to the average circulating levels of the gonadotropins (particularly follicle-stimulating hormone [FSH]) in a given population. As a result, it occurs slightly more frequently in women as they age or who undergo ovulation induction. It seems that serum FSH levels do vary among different ethnic groups: blacks have a higher level than whites, who in turn have a higher average serum FSH than Asians. The more FSH, the greater the probability of double ovulation in any given cycle.

DIAGNOSIS

There are three common ways to diagnose twins: physical exam, ultrasound, and maternal serum alpha-fetoprotein. Physical exam alone will fail to diagnose approximately 50% of twins. Although it may sound strange, in the days before ultrasound, obstetricians occasionally diagnosed twins by reaching inside the uterus to check on the placenta only to have it kick them. A surprise indeed!

While ultrasound is not completely accurate in diagnosing twins, its sensitivity and specificity is probably close to 99%, that is, of every 100 twin pregnancies, it will fail to diagnose 1. Therefore, ultrasound will miss one set of twins in every 10,000 pregnant Americans.

In a roundabout way, even maternal serum alpha-fetoprotein can aid with the diagnosis of twins. While it is primarily a screening tool for fetuses with neural tube defects, one cause of elevated levels (higher than 2.5 multiples of the median) can be twins. Part of the work-up of an initially elevated level is an ultrasound just for this purpose.

DIAGNOSIS OF ZYGOSITY

Determining the kinship between twins is often more than a matter of mere curiosity—it can have medical implications before and after birth. The first method that should be used is careful microscopic evaluation of the common membrane separating the pregnancies and using the following rules:

1. The thicker, outer membrane is the chorion, whereas the thinner membrane is the amnion.
2. Monochorionic twins are *always* monozygotic. They can either share or have separate amnionic membranes. Twins that share one amnion, while uncommon, are at extreme risk for cord accidents, and dual survival of monoamnionic twins is rare indeed. The identification of some membrane separating the fetuses during ultrasound is of more than just passing interest.
3. Dichorionic twins are usually, but *not* always, dizygotic. Identical twins will occasionally have separate chorions.

Thus, most identical twins can be diagnosed with certainty on the basis of the placenta, but the relationship between fraternal, same-sex twins cannot be proven similarly.

There are two other techniques that are commonly used to classify same-sex twins. The first is genetic blood typing in which a minimum number of proteins (usually eight) present on red blood cells are compared. If all eight proteins are identical, the probability of monozygosity is more than 95% (depending on the specific proteins). Of course, this probability rises with the number of proteins that are found to be shared between the siblings (as long as there are no differences).

A much cheaper method is to wait until the siblings are in their early teens and then ask their parents, "Are they as alike as two peas in a pod?" If both answer yes, the probability of monozygosity is greater than 90%.

MORBIDITY AND MORTALITY

The prenatal care for women with twin gestations differs somewhat from the standard protocol for those with singleton pregnancies. This is chiefly due to the fact that the perinatal mortality rate is four times higher than the singleton rate for the first twin and five times higher for the second twin. It is worthwhile to briefly review the causes for some of these adverse outcomes, because much of prenatal care is directed at averting them.

Prematurity

Approximately 50% of twin gestations deliver by 37 weeks. Prematurity is the biggest single factor in the high twin neonatal mortality rate and is a contributing factor in the majority of these deaths. The critical period seems to be delivery before 32 weeks with birth weights under 1500 g.

Intrauterine Growth Retardation

Definition. Another risk of multiple gestation is intrauterine growth retardation (IUGR). This is a difficult term to define, as will be seen. A better word for this idea is "malnourished fetus." This concept refers to the observation that some fetuses appear malnourished when born—thin and underweight for their length and gestational age. While these infants are usually easy to identify on visual inspection after birth, many authors have difficulty defining the term precisely. Probably the most widely used definition is a baby weighing under 2500 g who is also in the lowest 10th percentile weight group for his or her gestational age. Of course, this definition suggests that infants weighing over 2500 g cannot be classified as "growth retarded," yet some of them clearly appear to be malnourished.

Diagnosis. The antenatal diagnosis rests chiefly on ultrasound. With this technique, there are two types of IUGR identifiable: symmetric and asymmetric. Symmetric IUGR (the more severe form) occurs when both the body and the head have poor growth over serial scans. Asymmetric IUGR (the more common variety) may occur in mild cases of malnourishment because the head continues to grow at a more or less normal rate while the body has poor growth.

The ultrasound standards used for judging growth rate depend on the gestational age and the population studied. Biparietal diameters (width of the fetal head) and abdominal circumferences are most used to judge fetal growth, although other measurements such head circumference and femur length also may be of interest. There is debate about whether singleton growth curves and measurements can be appropriately applied to twins. Below-average volumes of amniotic fluid are also highly suggestive of IUGR, although the mechanism is unclear.

Treatment of IUGR is difficult at best. Bedrest, smoking cessation, and attention to maternal nutrition may be of modest benefit. Nonstress tests may be used in an effort to identify those malnourished fetuses at particular risk of demise. In extreme cases, premature delivery may be considered.

Risks. The diagnosis of IUGR carries with it an increased probability of short-term and long-term problems. As IUGR fetuses often have reduced amounts of amniotic fluid and relatively thin umbilical cords, the chances of compromise during labor are higher. Immediately after birth, hypothermia and hypoglycemia may emerge as problems due to decreased liver glycogen stores. Over the long term, these initially malnourished babies are thought to experience developmental delays and impaired school performance.

Twin-Twin Transfusion Syndrome

Peculiar to monozygotic twins, this problem occurs when the placental arteries of one twin empty into the veins of the other. As a result, one twin becomes polycythemic while the other becomes anemic. This potentially fatal problem can sometimes be diagnosed by ultrasound.

Additional Problems

Risks for the mother include an increased likelihood of hyperemesis gravidarum (severe nausea and vomiting); pregnancy-induced hypertension (preeclampsia); and postpartum hemorrhage (from uterine atony). Iron deficiency anemia is also more likely in mothers of twins. Other risks for the fetuses include an increased probability of congenital anomalies and malpresentation during labor.

PRENATAL CARE

Although recommendations vary greatly among obstetricians, an example of a prenatal treatment plan is the following:

1. Markedly decreased activity or bedrest in the third trimester
2. Weekly or biweekly prenatal visits after 24 weeks to check blood pressure and cervical dilatation
3. Monthly ultrasounds to measure growth in the late second trimester and beyond
4. Weekly nonstress testing at 34 to 36 weeks through delivery (earlier if IUGR is suspected)

These steps are designed to detect and avert the two largest threats to a twin gestation—prematurity and poor growth.

LABOR AND DELIVERY

The two chief areas of controversy in the delivery of twins are when to do a cesarean section for malpresentation and how to manage the delivery of the second twin if the first is delivered vaginally. It should be emphasized that there are several legitimate approaches.

As twins are almost invariably smaller at a given gestation, there is less concern about breech fetuses becoming entrapped within the maternal bony pelvis. However, premature breeches may still be better off with cesarean birth (see Chapter 18). One concern about delivering the first twin as a breech if the second twin is vertex is that, rarely, the chin of the first may "lock" with the chin of the second, impeding delivery. If the first fetus is head first, there is less concern about delivering the subsequent baby as a breech. Gestational age is also an important issue in deciding the route of delivery as very premature fetuses may experience more difficulties during labor. As a practical matter, many obstetricians (if not most) will get an abdominal x-ray at the outset of labor to more clearly identify the presentations and relative positioning of the twins.

With regard to delivery of the second twin, it was certainly true that morbidity and mortality rose with an increasing time interval between births in decades past. With the advent of electronic fetal monitoring, intervention at some arbitrary time limit seems less necessary. As the condition of the second twin can deteriorate rapidly, emergency cesarean section occasionally becomes necessary. Many obstetricians will try to leave the membranes intact around the second twin for as long as possible to reduce the chance of cord prolapse.

An alternative to cesarean section for rapid delivery of a breech second twin is a procedure known as "breech extraction" in which the feet of the fetus are grasped and brought out through the vagina. If the amniotic membranes are not ruptured by this time, most obstetricians prefer to leave them intact during a breech extraction. Breech extractions are often done under halothane anesthesia to permit uterine relaxation.

After both infants are born, uterine atony is the largest concern before and after delivery of the placenta. If bleeding is unusually brisk, the placentas can be manually removed. For heavy bleeding after the placentas have been delivered, bimanual uterine massage is usually immediately effective in helping the uterus contract. Of course, oxytocin and Methergine may also be beneficial.

18
CHAPTER

Breech

DEFINITION

There are two sets of definitions that are commonly encountered in any discussion of breeches, those referring to presentation and those referring to delivery.

Presentation

1. **Frank breech.** The presenting part of the fetus is the buttocks, and the legs are both flexed and parallel to the thorax (Fig. 18–1A).
2. **Complete breech.** The fetus has assumed a sitting position within the birth canal, but the buttocks are still the presenting part (Fig. 18–1B).
3. **Footling breech.** One or both feet are now inferior to the buttocks and will be the first part to deliver (Fig. 18–1C). This category is further divided into single-footling breech and double-footling breech.

Delivery

1. **Spontaneous breech.** The fetus is delivered without any assistance other than support of the body as it emerges.

Figure 18–1. Breech presentations. **A,** Frank breech presentation. **B,** Complete breech presentation. **C,** Footling breech presentation. (From Bonica, JJ: Principles and Practice of Obstetric Analgesia and Anesthesia. FA Davis, Philadelphia, 1967, p 1223, with permission.)

2. **Assisted breech or partial breech extraction.** The fetal arms and head are manipulated after delivery of the umbilicus. This route of delivery also describes the use of forceps for the head, although the use of forceps is often specifically mentioned in any description of the birth.
3. **Breech extraction.** This method of delivery involves grasping both feet and pulling the fetus through and out of the vagina. This is rarely done except possibly for rapid delivery of the second twin.

INCIDENCE AND CAUSE

At term, 3% to 4% of fetuses present as breeches. Of all breeches, 65% are frank versus 25% for footling and 10% for complete breech. Gestational age has a significant impact on the probability of breech presentation. In the mid-second trimester, roughly one fourth of fetuses are breech, whereas at 28 to 30 weeks, only 8% present this way. The percentage declines further as term approaches.

Why are some babies breech? No one really knows for sure. Theories include fundal implantation of the placenta (which only occurs in 7% of pregnancies) and some abnormality of fetal muscle tone. Some investigators have found motor abnormalities in children who were breech regardless of route of delivery. They speculate that the fetus was breech because of impaired ability to move within the uterus.

RISKS

Fetuses that are breech are exposed to greater risks during labor and delivery than those who emerge head first. This stems largely from two main problems: head entrapment and cord prolapse.

Head Entrapment

When a vertex fetus is too large for the maternal pelvis, progress in labor will ultimately stop. Whether delivery by cesarean is accomplished in minutes or in hours, the fetal condition does not usually change significantly without other complicating factors. The key difference in the delivery of a breech is that the largest part of the body, the head, is the last to deliver. Occasionally, the smaller thorax will deliver when the head will not. In such a circumstance, completing the delivery of the infant can be quite a challenge, as cesarean by this point is not usually a viable option (as the infant would literally have to be put back into the vagina and uterus). Because the baby cannot breathe while its oropharynx is still in the vagina and the umbilical cord is now compromised, the obstetrician has minutes rather than hours to accomplish delivery. The frightening feature of head entrapment is that it can be unpredictable, just as it is difficult to know which fetus and mother will experience cephalopelvic disproportion without a trial of labor. It is thought that proper selection of mothers for labor with breech presentations will keep this risk to a minimum.

Umbilical Cord Prolapse

With frank breech or vertex presentations, this obstetrical emergency only occurs in roughly 5 per 1000 labors. This risk rises to 50 per 1000 with complete breeches and 100 per 1000 for footling breeches. As a result, most obstetricians will consider labor and vaginal birth only for frank breeches.

MANAGEMENT

Ninety percent of all breech babies in the United States are delivered by cesarean section. With the well-recognized increased maternal morbidity and mortality rates for operative delivery, the key issue for breech delivery is, "Are there situations in which vaginal delivery poses no greater danger to the fetus than cesarean birth?" The literature suggests that there are indeed circumstances in which labor may be safely attempted, although there is still much controversy. Pragmatically, it is simply not possible to randomize 10,000 mothers with breech presentations and measure the outcome with different protocols.

Vaginal Birth

Space does not permit a meaningful review of the literature regarding this point. Listed below are some of the issues that are often considered in permitting mothers to labor.

1. **Gestational age.** Contrary to intuition, small, premature fetuses may actually have a higher risk from vaginal birth than those who are larger. Because the head to abdomen ratio is larger in the first half of the third trimester than in the second half, soft tissue entrapment poses a real threat. Many obstetricians advocate cesarean delivery for even frank breeches when less then 34 weeks.
2. **Frank breech.** Frank breeches seem most appropriate for vaginal birth because they do not have an increased risk of cord prolapse, as do complete and footling breeches.
3. **Estimated fetal weight.** Although neither ultrasound nor physical exam is entirely reliable, some suggest that a birth weight between 2500 and 3800 g has the least morbidity from vaginal birth.
4. **Prior deliveries.** Some advocate that primigravidas should not attempt labor with a breech, although the medical evidence supporting this contention is weak. This remains a very controversial issue.
5. **Oxytocin stimulation.** Some obstetricians will use oxytocin to stimulate or induce labor, but this too is controversial. Some argue that medical augmentation of labor may force a fetus with only a marginal fit through the pelvis. Of course, without oxytocin, some mothers who might otherwise have had a vaginal birth will require cesarean section. This would include those who do not go into labor after premature rupture of membranes

or those who require an induction of labor for medical reasons. Again, the view on oxytocin use during breech labor varies widely.

6. **X-ray pelvimetry.** Although largely discredited for predicting cephalopelvic disproportion with vertex presentations, x-ray measurement of bony landmarks may have some merit in those with breech. It can be used to eliminate those women with unusually small dimensions from undergoing a trial of labor. As with other issues in breech delivery, there is little consensus on its usefulness.

7. **Head hyperextension.** Five percent of breeches will have a "hyperextended head." This means that the head is flexed backward on the neck, also known as "star-gazing." This posture has been associated with increased probability of head entrapment or trauma to the cervical spine and is usually diagnosed by x-ray.

8. **Cervical exam.** The lower the breech is and the more dilated the cervix is at the start of labor, the more favorable the prognosis. Various investigators have tried to establish guidelines, but there is no universal agreement.

9. **Progress in labor.** Any vaginal trial of labor for breech presupposes that the labor progresses smoothly and that there is steady cervical dilatation and descent of the presenting part. Of course, electronic fetal monitoring is of value in helping to assure a favorable outcome.

The best candidates for labor are those who have spontaneous contractions with good cervical dilatation at the outset and medium-size babies. Ideally, the fetus should be a frank breech without head hyperexension. Since fetal posture is best demonstrated by x-ray and fetal weight is more accurately predicted by ultrasound, many obstetricians will obtain both studies at the outset of labor. Many authorities claim that vaginal birth poses no increased risk to the fetus and enhanced safety to the mother in "properly selected" cases.

Cesarean Section

As mentioned previously, 90% of breeches will be delivered by cesarean section. One unique consideration in the delivery of these infants is the orientation of the uterine incision. Hyperextension of the head and difficult delivery are still concerns if the uterine incision is too small. As a result, some advocate a lower cervical vertical incision to ensure an atraumatic birth. A large enough transverse incision may often suffice.

External Version

External version entails manipulating the fetus through the maternal abdominal wall in an effort to turn it to head first. There are several supportive studies in the medical literature, but the procedure has not received widespread acceptance. In general, the problems include separation of the placenta from the uterus, uterine rupture, fetal-maternal hemorrhage, and failure. Failure comes in two forms: an inability to turn the baby at the outset and a subsequent return to the breech position after an initially successful version. In the debate on external version, the disagreement does not concern the existence or nature of the various risks but their probability.

For those patients who seem to be appropriate candidates for version, the procedure is generally done in the hospital with provisions made for immediate cesarean section. Specifically, an IV is established and an operating room is prepared.

An ultrasound is used to guide the repositioning of the fetus, which is accomplished by steady, gentle hand-over-hand pressure. Agents that relax the uterus (such as ritodrine) are often administered prior to and during the procedure. Rh-negative mothers should probably receive Rh immune globulin.

19

CHAPTER

Preterm Labor

This chapter on preterm labor is meant to be only a thumbnail sketch of clinically relevant facts. Junior residents are encouraged to consult more experienced physicians whenever dealing with potential labor before term.

EPIDEMIOLOGY

Prematurity remains the leading cause of death for neonates without congenital anomalies. By definition, this is birth after 20 weeks' gestation and before 37 completed weeks (from the first day of the last menstrual period). In the United States, the incidence of preterm delivery is roughly 7% to 8%, and it is a factor in roughly three fourths of all neonatal deaths.

There are characteristics of a patient's history that may predict an increased risk for preterm labor. Unfortunately, such historical factors do not permit a very sensitive or specific forecast for prematurity. Examples of factors associated with subsequent early labor include a history of preterm labor in a prior pregnancy, smoking more than half a pack a day, DES exposure in utero, and history of a cone biopsy (removal of the central portion of the cervix to detect premalignant and malignant conditions). Certain complications of pregnancy have also been thought to increase the risk of preterm labor. These include uterine anomalies, pyelonephritis, advanced cervical dilatation, excess amniotic fluid, and, of course, twins.

DIAGNOSIS

The diagnosis of preterm labor rests heavily on its definition: uterine contractions leading to progressive cervical dilatation and effacement before 37 completed weeks of pregnancy. Although the definition seems clear enough, there are certain practical difficulties in making this diagnosis. First, the early contractions of preterm labor may not be as distinct to the patient as active labor at term. Many will describe their contractions as "the baby balling up," back pain, or intestinal cramping. Indeed, some patients may have diarrhea at the time they begin their labor so that their presentation may be quite confused.

Because the success of intervention steadily declines with advancing dilatation, there is some pressure on the physician to decide rapidly. On the other hand, as the intervention often includes strict bedrest for the rest of pregnancy and a complete cessation of work, the obstetrician is also inclined to avoid overdiagnosing the condition. Finally, there are some patients who will have regular contractions for a few hours at a time or even days who do not have cervical change and who will ultimately deliver at term. Although a minority, this group of women further complicates making an accurate diagnosis.

The differential diagnosis of preterm labor includes disorders of the uterus, bowel, urinary tract, and even the abdominal musculature. Separation of the placenta from the uterus can indeed cause contractions and even labor, but it should be considered as a separate entity as it can cause immediate fetal and even maternal demise (see Chapter 20). Other disorders of the uterus that can be confused with preterm labor include the pain of degenerating fibroids and rarely, fetal movement. Intestinal disorders, including appendicitis, spastic bowel, and constipation, can mimic early preterm labor. Indeed, the uterus may actually contract occasionally in response to these disorders, but premature delivery is not a common outcome in these circumstances.

Cystitis, pyelonephritis, and ureteral stones can all mimic the symptoms of preterm labor. As with the bowel disorders, these conditions can actually be associated with uterine contractions, and pyelonephritis is thought to be a risk factor for preterm delivery. Finally, some patients will present with episodic lower abdominal pain that will prove to be a result of some strain within or trauma to the abdominal wall.

In practice, any change in cervical dilatation or effacement in the presence of uterine contractions may be considered evidence of labor before term. Patients who present before 37 completed weeks with contractions and who are 2 cm or more dilated or more than 80% effaced are highly likely to be in labor. It is not unusual for multiparous patients to be 2 cm dilated in the middle of the third trimester, but those with contractions should usually be treated. Finally, regular contractions (eight or so in an hour) in the presence of ruptured membranes may also be regarded as labor, although the management may be different than when the membranes are intact.

TREATMENT

Treatment consists primarily of two modalities: bedrest and medication.

Bedrest

There are a variety of studies suggesting that bedrest is beneficial in either forestalling labor or helping to interrupt established labor in association with medication. As none of these studies are prospective randomized trials and many of them pertain to twins, the precise efficacy of bedrest is still uncertain. Nevertheless, virtually all obstetricians will incorporate rigorous bedrest in the long-term treatment of anyone with preterm labor.

IV hydration is often recommended as an early form of intervention, prior to initiating pharmacological agents. While I have seen many apparent successes with hydration alone, it may be that uterine activity ceases with the passage of a few hours rather than through volume expansion.

Pharmacological Agents

There are two main classes of drugs used to treat uterine contractions: beta sympathomimetics and magnesium. Other agents such as ethanol and prostaglandin inhibitors may have some benefit in inhibiting labor but are not as widely used. Ethanol has very unpleasant side effects, and the prostaglandin inhibitors simply have not been studied as much. There are also lingering concerns about their safety for the fetus.

Beta Sympathomimetics. So named because they preferentially stimulate the beta-adrenergic receptors, the two drugs most commonly used are ritodrine (Yutopar) and terbutaline. These agents are preferred because they show some predilection for $beta_2$ activity versus $beta_1$.

The $beta_2$ responses include decreased smooth muscle tone in the uterus, bronchioles, and vasculature. Urinary output is also decreased, and both glycogenolysis and insulin release are increased. As these drugs do have some $beta_1$ activity, they will also increase pulse rate. Pulmonary edema has been reported in patients on beta sympathomimetics. While an uncommon complication, it seems unpredictable and not necessarily related to dosage.

The side effects of beta sympathomimetics can be predicted from their physiological action. Decreased diastolic blood pressure (and faintness or dizziness); pounding and rapid heart rate; and an increase in serum glucose with a corresponding decrease in potassium are all prominent features of treatment. In addition, many patients will actually develop a tremor or jitteriness. The net result is that some patients may become quite uncomfortable at the higher doses of medication.

There are no known long-term ill effects from intrauterine exposure to beta sympathomimetics. The drugs do cause an increase in the fetal heart rate. As might be expected, neonates exposed to these agents during labor have temporary hypoglycemia, neonatal ileus, and hypotension.

Sample Ritodrine Protocol

1. Establish that preterm labor is occurring and obtain maternal medical history. Magnesium (see below) may be a better choice in the event of maternal diabetes, bleeding, or heart condition.
2. Obtain CBC with platelets, and serum electrolytes and glucose. A pretreatment ECG may be warranted to help evaluate any subsequent

chest pain or cardiac irregularities. Fluid balance should be carefully monitored. Occasionally a Foley catheter is of benefit.

3. Begin an IV drip and then start the medication at 50 to 100 µg/min. A computerized infusion pump should be used.

4. Increase the dose by 50 µg/min every 15 minutes until contractions are fewer than four per hour or to maximum dose of 350 µg/min.

5. Output and vitals should be checked frequently. In particular, once a maternal pulse of 140 is achieved, it is wise not to increase the dose further, regardless of the success of labor inhibition.

6. Maintain steady-state dosing for 6 to 12 hours. As a rule, fetal monitoring is continuous, and the patient remains observed in labor and delivery until she is stable on oral medication.

7. Wean to oral medication by giving 10 to 20 mg of ritodrine orally 1 hour prior to stopping the IV medication. Follow-up with 10 to 20 mg of oral ritodrine every 2 to 4 hours as necessary. The oral dosing is determined empirically by observing the patient in the hospital for at least 1 or 2 days.

8. Hypokalemia and elevated glucoses while on therapy are not treated unless they represent pre-existing conditions or are abnormal in the extreme.

Magnesium Sulfate. The mechanism of action is thought to be related to calcium antagonism. That is, it seems that magnesium decreases the intracellular free calcium necessary for smooth muscle contraction. Unfortunately, magnesium has this effect on all muscle. At 4 mEq/mL, deep tendon reflexes tend to be decreased, whereas at levels of 12 mEq/mL, respiratory depression occurs as well as cardiac impairment. At intermediate levels, patients may experience flushing, headaches, and nystagmus. In practice, one of the most debilitating side effects is a difficult-to-describe dysphoria in which many feel as though they are trapped within a dark cloud.

As with the beta sympathomimetics, there are no known ill long-term effects of magnesium on the fetus. (Occasionally, a decrease in muscle tone may be noted initially if the neonate was born while the mother was being treated with large doses of magnesium, as it crosses the placenta.)

Sample Magnesium Protocol

1. Follow steps 1 and 2 in the ritodrine protocol above. An ECG is less necessary for those on magnesium, although it might be helpful to confirm a normal calcium level before starting the drug. As with ritodrine, urine output should be closely watched as magnesium levels can rise in the face of oliguria.

2. Give a loading dose of 4 g over 10 to 20 minutes and then infuse magnesium at the rate of 1 to 3 g/h. A computerized infusion pump should be used. The dosage of magnesium should not exceed 4 g/h because toxic levels may be reached.

3. Increase the dose in $1/2$-g quantities every 15 minutes until the contractions are four or fewer per hour.

4. The dose should probably not be increased in the presence of significant nystagmus. If the respiratory rate slows on magnesium, stop the drug at least temporarily.

5. There is debate about the usefulness of checking magnesium levels, because the clinical status of the patient is a usually reasonably reliable indicator of drug level. Nevertheless, it is not unreasonable to check the serum magnesium every 6 to 12 hours. Keep in mind that it takes hours for magnesium to equilibrate in

the bloodstream. Both respiratory rate and deep tendon reflexes should be carefully monitored, although the deep tendon reflexes are more sensitive.

6. After uterine relaxation has been achieved, some obstetricians will switch to oral beta sympathomimetics. There have been reports of oral magnesium supplementation, but this requires very large quantities of medicine to achieve significant blood levels.

Contraindications to Tocolysis

There are some conditions in which the risk to the fetus and to the mother is less with a preterm birth than with tocolysis. As an example, with extreme maternal hemorrhage, it is probably more prudent to accomplish delivery rather than to delay it. Sometimes magnesium is a more appropriate choice of drug than ritodrine. Maternal diabetes, heart conditions, and bleeding are all circumstances in which magnesium might be preferred. Using tocolytics in women with ruptured membranes remains controversial and seems to be less effective.

Follow-up

Patients at high risk for preterm labor or who are already on medication for it are usually placed on complete bedrest at home. There is some thought that sexual intercourse may hasten labor as a result of the prostaglandins in semen. The notion that orgasm may precipitate labor has not been confirmed in the medical literature.

Patients are advised to have weekly office visits during which the cervix is checked. Those who have changed from one week to the next can be monitored for several hours (usually in labor and delivery) to be sure that they are not actively contracting. Tocolytic agents can be stopped at the beginning of the 37th week.

PROGRESSION OF PRETERM LABOR

Once labor is well established, tocolysis usually fails. Specifically, few patients who dilate to 4 cm or beyond with documentable contractions are going to respond to intervention. If delivery appears inevitable, the medications should be stopped and the pediatricians should be notified. The time course of preterm labor is notoriously variable, and the cervix does not need to dilate as completely to permit the passage of a premature fetus. Keep in mind that there is an increased incidence of breech before term and that the smaller breeches may be better off with cesarean delivery.

THE NEWBORN PREMATURE INFANT

Morbidity and Mortality

The probability of survival for a given neonate depends both on gestational age as well as birth weight. A newborn at 26 weeks who weighs 900 g is more likely to survive than one who weighs 700 g. Conversely, the 700-g fetus who is actually 28 weeks has a better prognosis than one at 26 weeks with the same weight.

Assuming an average weight, the approximate probability of survival at 26 weeks is on the order of 30%. At 32 weeks, more than 90% of those delivered will live. These statistics have been improving steadily over the last decade.

Of course, another issue is the quality of life for survivors. This remains somewhat controversial. As gestational age increases, the long-term deficits among survivors markedly decreases. The majority of those delivered at and beyond 32 weeks are not handicapped and even most delivered before this time will grow to lead normal lives.

By and large, there are at least six major threats to the premature neonate:

1. **Respiratory distress.** This is discussed below.
2. *Patent ductus areteriosus.* Particularly in very premature infants, the ductus arteriosus may fail to close promptly, resulting in at least a temporary left-to-right shunt that can result in congestive heart failure. In extreme cases, prostaglandin inhibitors or surgical ligature may be necessary.
3. **Intraventricular hemorrhage and neurological deficits.** The cerebral blood vessels seem particularly fragile in premature infants. The veins are prone to tears, which can lead to significant intracranial hemorrhage. In more severe cases, the blood can leak into the ventricles, which may interfere with absorption of intraventricular fluid and further compromise neural tissue. "Traumatic" birth has traditionally been thought to be a cause, but it is becoming increasingly evident that preterm fetuses are prone to this problem no matter what the route of delivery. It should also be noted that there is an association between prematurity, low birth weight, and cerebral palsy, although the etiology is unclear.
4. **Hyperbilirubinemia.** This may become a problem in preterm infants because the liver may not have matured enough to fully metabolize bilirubin in the first few days of life.

With high enough levels sustained over a period of time, bilirubin toxicity can occur, resulting in brain damage. In mild to moderate elevations of bilirubin, exposure of the newborn to ultraviolet light assists the metabolism of bilirubin. In more severe cases, exchange transfusions may be required in which the neonate's blood is removed and replaced with donor blood with a low bilirubin content.

5. **Sepsis.** Premature infants are less able to fend off bacteria and can succumb rapidly to infections that full-term infants would otherwise survive. Diagnosing sepsis in these infants can also be quite difficult as they show few signs or symptoms of illness until the infection is quite advanced. Pneumonia and meningitis are infections of particular concern.

6. **Feeding difficulties.** As can be imagined, nutrition of the premature infant is no simple matter. Not only are his or her nutritional requirements not fully known but also the gastrointestinal tract is frequently not prepared to be the primary source of nutrient processing. As an example, coordination between swallowing and respiration does not reliably occur before 32 to 34 weeks, and aspiration of oral intake is a problem before this time. Frequently, gavage feeding (through a tube that passes through the mouth or nose into the stomach) is necessary. In extremely ill neonates, hyperalimentation may be required.

RESPIRATORY DISTRESS SYNDROME

One of the biggest problems facing the premature infant is respiration. The major obstacle to sustained spontaneous respiration is the absence of surfactant—a lipoprotein mixture that decreases the surface tension within the lungs. Without surfactant, the lungs are relatively stiff and inflexible, leading to rapid tiring of the newborn. Without mechanical assistance, many would succumb.

At 34 to 36 weeks, most fetuses begin producing surfactant in significant quantities. The probability of respiratory distress syndrome (RDS) can be predicted while the fetus is still in utero from measuring lipoproteins within the amnionic fluid (through amniocentesis). By measuring the ratio of phosphatidylcholine (lecithin) to sphingomyelin (the L/S ratio) the likelihood of RDS can be estimated. For those with an L/S of 2:1 or more, RDS occurs less than 2% of the time. Those with a ratio of less than 2:1 have up to a 50% chance of developing the disease. As a practical matter, the L/S ratio can help obstetricians decide whether or not to use drugs to inhibit labor. For instance, in a patient at 35 weeks who is contracting, a rapidly obtained L/S ratio can serve as a guide to how vigorous an effort should be made to stop labor.

Another issue encountered in obstetrics is the use of glucocorticoids to enhance fetal lung maturity. There is some evidence that steroids given 2 to 7 days in advance of delivery between 28 and 32 weeks' gestation may promote surfactant production. There is controversy over exactly when to use this approach, as few can reliably predict that delivery will be "2 to 7 days away." Although there are no known ill effects of this medication on the fetus, the experience with administering DES to pregnant patients has made some physicians hesitant to use steroids except in very limited circumstances. The risk of pulmonary edema in patients being treated with beta sympathomimetics may be increased with the concomitant use of glucocorticoids.

Exogenously introduced surfactant became widely available in the early 1990s. An aerosol spray, it is dispersed throughout the lungs via intubation and mechanical ventilation. It has revolutionized care in the neonatal intensive care unit and has made RDS almost an historical curiosity. The availability of surfactant will probably change obstetrical management over time, particularly in terms of preterm premature rupture of membranes, but it has yet to do so.

PRETERM PREMATURE RUPTURE OF THE MEMBRANES

Also known as preterm PROM, this complication occurs in roughly 1% of pregnancies. PROM refers to the amniotic membranes breaking before the onset of labor, whether at term or before. Of course, preterm PROM occurs before 37 completed weeks' gestation.

Complications

The two chief complications of preterm PROM are labor and uterine infection. Roughly 80% of pregnant patients will spontaneously labor within 1 week of this event. Of course, the vast majority of those who break the membranes before term will be destined to delivery prematurely. Because many of these patients will spontaneously dilate and efface in the apparent absence of contractions, the diagnosis of labor can be quite difficult to make.

Infection is perhaps even more of a concern, as it can definitely jeopardize maternal well being. Those who develop a uterine infection while the fetus remains inside (chorioamnionitis) can become septic and deteriorate quite rapidly, although this is not often the case. The signs and symptoms of chorioamnionitis include an elevated maternal temperature (anything over 99.4°F should be regarded suspiciously); fetal or maternal tachycardia; and uterine contractions or tenderness.

Known chorioamnionitis is a contraindication to tocolysis. Prolonging the pregnancy under these circumstances increases both maternal and fetal risk, at least in extreme cases. Fortunately, tocolysis is rarely successful in those with chorioamnionitis. When it is difficult to distinguish between labor and infection, some obstetricians will use magnesium to stall for time until the diagnosis becomes more clear. As ritodrine raises both the maternal and fetal pulse, it can cloud the issue.

Many advocate obtaining serial white blood cell counts to assist in detection of chorioamnionitis. Although not a bad idea, a significantly elevated white count is usually a late finding. Maternal pulse and temperature seem to be the most sensitive.

Diagnosis

In the initial assessment of preterm PROM, several steps should be taken immediately. First, the diagnosis should be confirmed by sterile speculum exam, nitrazine paper, and the finding of a ferning pattern of the fluid as it dries under magnification. If the diagnosis is either confirmed or suspected, a digital cervical exam should be avoided unless delivery is imminent (within hours), as this has been linked to an increased probability of chorioamnionitis. Finally, cervical cultures for betahemolytic strep, gonorrhea, and possibly chlamydia should be obtained, because the presence of these organisms is associated with increased neonatal morbidity. At the least, mothers with preterm PROM should be placed on bedrest. Some obstetricians will have the patient observed in the hospital for several days (if not longer), depending on the patient's reliability.

20

CHAPTER

Third Trimester Bleeding

Third trimester bleeding can result from something as trivial as a localized vaginal infection or it can be the harbinger of hemorrhage and death. In the nonpregnant state, the uterus receives approximately 1% of cardiac output. In the third trimester, it receives 20% of an increased cardiac output. Uterine bleeding in the third trimester can be quite impressive. This chapter deals primarily with evaluation of the hemodynamically stable patient.

For those patients who arrive at the hospital literally pouring out blood, there are two immediate objectives of treatment: fluid replacement and delivery. Transfusions and fluid serve as a temporizing measure until delivery can be accomplished. Ultimately, the one sure way to stop severe obstetrical hemorrhage is to deliver the fetus and remove the placenta. Fortunately, patients rarely present with hemorrhage and hypovolemic shock. There are usually smaller bleeds that may serve as warnings.

EVALUATION OF A PATIENT WITH THIRD TRIMESTER BLEEDING

Third trimester bleeding occurs in approximately 4% of patients. About half will have an inconsequential cause, whereas the remainder will have either placenta previa or an abruption. There are two diagnostic clues to discerning the cause of the bleeding: the history and physical.

History

Ask about prior episodes, abdominal pain, uterine contractions, and recent intercourse.

Examination

Assessment of uterine contractions and tenderness is critical. Electronic fetal monitoring should be initiated to detect potential compromise. Finally, a gentle speculum exam should be performed in an effort to distinguish cervical from uterine bleeding (often difficult). During visualization of the cervix, some assessment should be made of dilation.

A digital cervical exam should not be done until the placental location is established by ultrasound. Prior to the widespread use of this test, it was common to examine patients with third trimester bleeding with the "double set-up examination." This entailed an exam in the cesarean section room with the patient prepped for an immediate cesarean section in case the examiner disrupted placental integrity in those with a previa. With the high accuracy of ultrasound, this is now rarely necessary.

There is some controversy about whether a

speculum exam should be done before knowing the location of the placenta. Some argue that the speculum can be as traumatic as a digital exam. It is certainly reasonable to do the ultrasound first if the situation permits.

Other

If an ultrasound has not recently identified the location of the placenta, one should be obtained. The prenatal Pap smear should be double checked. As part of the evaluation, a CBC should be obtained along with a coagulation profile (PT, PTT, fibrin degradation products, platelet count, and fibrinogen). For any patient who seems to have uterine bleeding, some blood should be cross-matched. The number of units that should be standing by depends on the circumstances, but 4 U is often a good place to start.

DIFFERENTIAL DIAGNOSIS

1. **Contact bleeding.** As the cervix is more vascular during pregnancy, intercourse can rupture a cervical blood vessel, resulting in bleeding that can be impressive. This diagnosis is made when suggested by the history and other causes are excluded.
2. **Cervical inflammation.** Occasionally, vaginal infections will cause the cervix to spontaneously bleed, although the quantity of blood is usually small. Again, other causes should be excluded.
3. **Cervical effacement and dilatation.** Occasionally, vaginal bleeding may be the presenting complaint of someone experiencing labor.

Usually, bleeding during labor will be accompanied by the passage of cervical mucus, although not always. Rarely, the bleeding may be brisk enough to suggest other causes.

4. **Placenta previa.** This refers to the placenta "preceding" the fetus and actually covering the cervix. See the next section.

5. **Placental abruption.** Premature separation of the placenta from the uterine wall is known as abruption. This is discussed in a later section.

6. **Other.** Coagulation disorders and cervical cancer are very uncommon causes of third trimester bleeding. The initial labs should help suggest a coagulation disorder if one exists. Checking the prenatal Pap and visualizing the cervix can usually eliminate cancer as a cause.

PLACENTA PREVIA

Prior to the past century, placenta previa had roughly a 30% maternal mortality rate and was almost universally fatal for the fetus.

Incidence

Placenta previa occurs roughly once in every 250 pregnancies. Its incidence increases significantly as parity rises. Although a "low-lying" placenta may be visualized relatively frequently in the second trimester, 90% of these resolve and do not pose problems as the uterus grows. Placenta previa is somewhat more common in those who have had multiple abortions. The risk of recurrence in subsequent pregnancies is roughly 4% to 8%.

Diagnosis

The characteristic presentation of placenta previa is painless vaginal bleeding in the late second trimester or in the third trimester. The first episode of bleeding is most common near 34 weeks' gestation. Sometimes, placenta previa will be associated with either an abruption or labor. The presence of contractions does not exclude this diagnosis.

There are several definitions of placenta previa worth reviewing. A complete previa means that the placenta is entirely covering the cervix. With a partial previa, the placenta covers only part of the cervical os. In a marginal previa, the placenta just reaches the cervix. Finally, a low lying placenta is one near, but not abutting, the cervical opening.

Treatment

Treatment consists of two approaches: delivery by cesarean and delay of delivery for as long as possible. However, the longer the pregnancy continues, the higher the risk of major hemorrhage. As a result, it is common practice to perform an amniocentesis for the L/S ratio at 36 weeks. Fetuses with a low probability of respiratory distress syndrome are then promptly delivered. This practice may start to change with the widespread availability of exogenous surfactant.

Most patients with placenta previa will have repetitive episodes of bleeding. As a result, once the diagnosis of previa is made, they will be kept at bedrest for the remainder of the pregnancy, often in the hospital. Although this can be quite expensive, it is nearly impossible to predict the timing or volume of the next bleed. As a consequence, most obstetricians will have 2 to 4 U of blood typed and cross-matched at all times. Some will also have a large bore IV line maintained continuously until delivery.

The chief method of buying time for the fetus other than bedrest is through maternal blood transfusions. Again, because bleeding tends to be recurrent and unpredictable, most physicians will try to keep the maternal hemoglobin above some arbitrary value. Transfusing to keep the hemoglobin at 10 g or above is the figure most often cited in the literature. This practice helps to assure adequate oxygenation for the fetus and some protection of the mother in the event of future blood loss.

When bleeding episodes do occur in the hospital, it is wise to transfer the mother from the antepartum floor to labor and delivery for fetal monitoring and close observation. For anything but the most insignificant bleeding, preparations should be made for cesarean section. Patients with placenta previa may have to be moved to and from labor and delivery several times during the pregnancy.

Even with the strategy of bedrest in the hospital, blood transfusions, and cesarean birth, a good outcome cannot be guaranteed. The maternal mortality rate with this condition is at least somewhat increased, although it is less than 1%. The perinatal mortality rate is higher, on the order of 10% to 15%.

Complications

There are several adverse outcomes that are associated with placenta previa. Intrauterine growth retardation is thought to be more common, and the incidence of congenital anomalies is roughly doubled. One particularly fearsome complication is that of placenta accreta—a condition in which the placenta has abnormally attached to the myometrium. The result is that there is no smooth cleavage plane, and it is impossible to entirely separate the placenta from the uterine wall. As a result, the placental site continues to bleed following delivery. Often, the only cure for this problem is removal of the uterus, as less drastic measures seldom succeed in achieving hemostasis. Placenta accreta is a particular concern if the previa occurs in a patient with a prior cesarean, but it can also occur in a normally located placenta.

ABRUPTION

Abruption refers to premature separation of the placenta from the uterine wall. This separation can be partial or complete. A clinically evident abruption poses a risk to both mother and fetus.

Incidence

Abruption is thought to complicate roughly 1% of all pregnancies. Hypertension, cigarette smoking, and even trauma (severe) all predispose to placental separation. Those who have had a prior abruption are at increased risk for recurrence (roughly 6%). Abruption accounts for approximately 10% to 15% of all perinatal deaths. The risk to the fetus comes from anoxia, exsanguination, or premature delivery.

Diagnosis

The diagnosis of abruption is dependent on the history and physical. Ultrasound and lab studies can suggest the diagnosis, but the patient's presentation is key. The classic signs and symptoms of abruption are vaginal bleeding, uterine tenderness, and contractions. Of course, in early or mild cases, some patients will only have one of these problems at the outset.

Ultrasound is useful for excluding placenta previa but cannot reliably confirm the diagnosis of placental separation. A drop in hemoglobin or decrease in coagulability also suggests the diagnosis, but again, it is the patient's signs and symptoms that are key. Disseminated intravascular coagulation (DIC) occurs in less than 10% of cases and is more common in those with fetal demise or excessive blood loss.

Management

As with all cases of third trimester bleeding, establish first that the mother is hemodynamically stable by noting pulse, blood pressure, skin color, mentation, and the like. Then establish heart tones and begin electronic fetal monitoring. Volume replacement, transfusion, and immediate delivery (by cesarean) are appropriate for mothers with continued bleeding or for fetal distress. In mild abruptions with mothers who are stable with no evidence of fetal distress, bedrest and observation may be appropriate.

DIC is one of the most serious complications of an abruption. DIC is characterized by spontaneous bleeding from places such as the nose or the IV site. Although the treatment of this complication is beyond the scope of this book, the approach usually consists of massive blood transfusions, immediate delivery, and occasionally, the use of a MAST suit. Once the fetus and placenta are delivered, the illness usually resolves spontaneously, although patients can become quite ill in the meantime.

21

CHAPTER

Forceps Delivery and Vacuum Extraction

The original use for forceps was to extract a dead baby from its mother. This situation was a desperate one, as safe cesarean section has only been available for the past century. Failure to extract the fetus would mean almost certain maternal death. Of course, for the past several centuries, forceps have been more commonly used to assist with difficult births. Currently, forceps are used to shorten labor whenever the mother or fetus might benefit. They are no longer used when a difficult birth is anticipated, as most obstetricians will resort to abdominal delivery in these circumstances.

DEFINITIONS

The definitions below are taken from an American College of Obstetricians and Gynecologists committee opinion that was published in February, 1988. The cervix has to be completely dilated before forceps can be applied.

Outlet Forceps

There are several conditions that need to be fulfilled for a delivery to qualify as outlet forceps. First, the sagittal suture has to be in the anterior-posterior plane. This means that the fetus is either direct occiput anterior or direct occiput posterior—no rotation beyond 45° is necessary. Second, the scalp is visible without separating the labia. With these criterion, application of forceps qualifies as outlet forceps.

Low Forceps

This entails the use of forceps when the leading part of the fetal skull is at station +2 or more. By definition, low forceps can involve rotation of more than 45°. Station in this case refers to the distance (in centimeters) between the leading portion of the fetal skull and the maternal ischial spines. A more abstract definition of station is the relationship of the biparietal diameter to the pelvic inlet. Of course, this cannot be measured directly, and the preceding definition may be of more practical use.

Midforceps

A midforceps delivery describes application of the forceps when the fetal skull is higher than +2 station or when significant rotation is required.

High Forceps

No longer done under any circumstances, this refers to the delivery of the "unengaged" fetus (above 0 station) by forceps.

INDICATIONS

The indications for forceps delivery are the shortening of labor to benefit either the mother or the fetus. With electronic fetal monitoring, obstetricians are less compelled to deliver the fetus after some arbitrary length of time has elapsed than they might have been previously. One of the more common reasons for using forceps is maternal exhaustion. Other circumstances include fetal distress or maternal heart disease.

There is controversy over the safety of mid-forceps deliveries, particularly those requiring significant rotation. Some information published in the medical literature suggests an increased morbidity rate for fetuses delivered by this technique. Because a meaningful prospective randomized trial would be impossible to conduct, the issue may never be resolved. Some of the information comes from deliveries that occurred 20 years ago or more, and it is particularly difficult to apply those experiences to current practice. Several decades ago, it was routine to deliver patients by forceps from relatively high stations while the mother was given general anesthesia. As this type of intervention was much more aggressive than current practice, data from this experience simply do not reflect more recent outcomes accurately. Nothing suggests any increased morbidity from low or outlet forceps delivery.

TECHNIQUE

Before applying forceps, the patient's bladder should be emptied and the fetal position con-

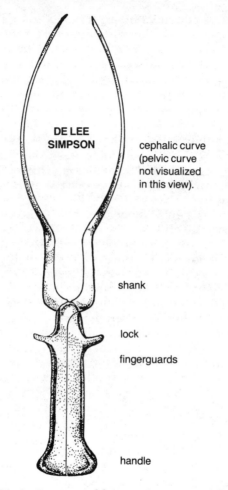

Figure 21–1. Features of forceps (DeLee modification of Simpson forceps). Note that pelvic curve is not visualized in this view. (Adapted from Dennen, PC: Dennen's Forceps Deliveries, ed 3. FA Davis, Philadelphia, 1989, p 18, with permission.)

firmed. A pudendal block provides some benefit, but regional anesthesia is often preferable. After the delivery, a special effort should be made to inspect the vaginal walls for lacerations, particularly near the ischial spines. Occasionally, the delivery may prove to be more difficult than anticipated, in which case a cesarean section may be performed.

The forceps themselves can be described by four features (Fig. 21–1). The blade is the portion that actually grasps the fetus. Its cephalic curve corresponds to the shape of the fetal head while the pelvic curve conforms to the general architecture of the maternal pelvis. Blades can be solid or hollowed out for a more firm application. The second feature of forceps is the shank, which connects the blade to the lock and handle. The shanks can either overlap or be separate. The lock is the portion that actually holds the two branches together. Finally, the handle is the part that is grasped by the obstetrician.

Figure 21–2. Manual method of axis traction. (From Dennen, PC: Dennen's Forceps Deliveries, ed 3. FA Davis, Philadelphia, 1989, p 57, with permission.)

The method of application depends on the forceps and position of the fetus. In general, the blades are designed for application to the sides of the fetal head rather than from front to back. It is often helpful to apply traction during a contraction while having the mother push at the same time (Fig. 21–2). With low forceps or midforceps, the delivery often takes several contractions to accomplish.

VACUUM EXTRACTION

The principles for forceps delivery also apply to vacuum extraction. With this technique, a cup is placed on the fetal scalp and suction is applied to create an airtight seal. The suction may be provided by either an electric or hand-powered pump. When using the vacuum, care must be taken to be sure that maternal tissues are not included in the application. With the vacuum devices commonly used today, the seal is readily broken if too much force is applied. In comparison to forceps, the vacuum extractor provides less traction but also less chance of vaginal lacerations.

Epilogue

At the time of this second edition, I have been in private practice for 6 years. These years have provided me with an interesting perspective on my residency experience and career choice.

I went into obstetrics and gynecology for four main reasons. This surgical specialty offers an opportunity for decisive intervention and cure. It also focuses heavily on preventive medicine in terms of contraception, sexually transmitted disease detection and prevention, and prenatal care. By and large, the delivery of babies is a very happy experience. Perhaps the most important reason for choosing this specialty is the ability to establish long-term contact with individual patients. Although much of medicine becomes routine and dull given enough time, the "normal vaginal birth in bed 120B" has more meaning if it is Mrs. Smith whom I have known for several years.

Malpractice crisis and increased government interference notwithstanding, I have found the four reasons above to be largely valid. Although I am not particularly good at remembering names and faces, I find it particularly satisfying when I can link a name on the phone or the appointment list with someone I know. This is not often achievable in a residency program where contact with a particular patient is limited by the length of a rotation.

I do not like getting out of bed in the middle of the night any more than the next person, but I still get a thrill out of deliveries. There is something marvelous about witnessing the first moments of a new life. Perhaps it will help medical students and junior residents to know that, at least for me, the struggle was worth it.

Appendix

COMMONLY USED ABBREVIATIONS

AFP. Alpha fetoprotein
AROM. Artificial rupture of membranes
BPD. Biparietal diameter
BPM. Beats per minute
CPD. Cephalopelvic disproportion
EDC. Estimated date of confinement
FHT. Fetal heart tones
HPI. History of present illness
IUFD. Intrauterine fetal demise
IUGR. Intrauterine growth retardation
IUPC. Intrauterine pressure catheter
LMP. Last menstrual period
LTV. Long-term variability
NST. Nonstress test
NTD. Neural tube defect
PMH. Past medical history
PROM. Premature rupture of membranes
ROS. Review of systems
SROM. Spontaneous rupture of membranes
STV. Short-term variability

Index

An "f" following a page number indicates a figure; a "t" indicates a table.